LOCAL
FOOD

LOCAL
FOOD

HOW TO MAKE IT HAPPEN
IN YOUR COMMUNITY

Tamzin Pinkerton & Rob Hopkins

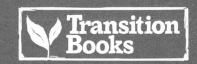

Transition Books

First published in 2009 by

Transition Books
an imprint of Green Books
www.transitionbooks.net

Green Books
Foxhole, Dartington
Totnes, Devon TQ9 6EB
www.greenbooks.co.uk

Design by Stephen Prior

Illustration on page 7 © Jennifer Johnson

Image on page 11: all reasonable efforts have been
made to obtain copyright permission for the
reproduction of this photograph. If the copyright
holder is able to contact us we would be happy to
give credit in the next edition.

Printed in the UK by Cambrian Printers.
The text paper is made from 100% recycled post-
consumer waste, and the covers from 75% recycled
material.

DISCLAIMER: The advice in this book is believed to
be correct at the time of printing, but the authors and
the publishers accept no liability for actions inspired
by this book.

ISBN 978 1 900322 43 0

CONTENTS

Dedications   8

Acknowledgements   9

Foreword by Rosie Boycott   10

Introduction by Rob Hopkins   11

Chapter 1   The local food movement   20
Chapter 2   The Great Reskilling   35
Chapter 3   Home garden growing in the community   47
Chapter 4   Allotment provision and gardening for community groups   56
Chapter 5   Garden shares   71
Chapter 6   Community gardens   79
Chapter 7   Community orchards   91
Chapter 8   Community Supported Agriculture   102
Chapter 9   Farmers' markets   114
Chapter 10   Food cooperatives   123
Chapter 11   Local food guides and directories   132
Chapter 12   School projects on local food   141
Chapter 13   Local food events   150
Chapter 14   Expanding local food projects   158
Chapter 15   Yet more inspired ideas   164
Chapter 16   The local food project and beyond   175

References   185

Resources   190

Index   211

"We cannot be free if our food and its sources are controlled by someone else. The condition of the passive consumer of food is not a democratic condition. One reason to eat responsibly is to live free."

Wendell Berry, 'The Pleasures of Eating' in *What Are People For?*

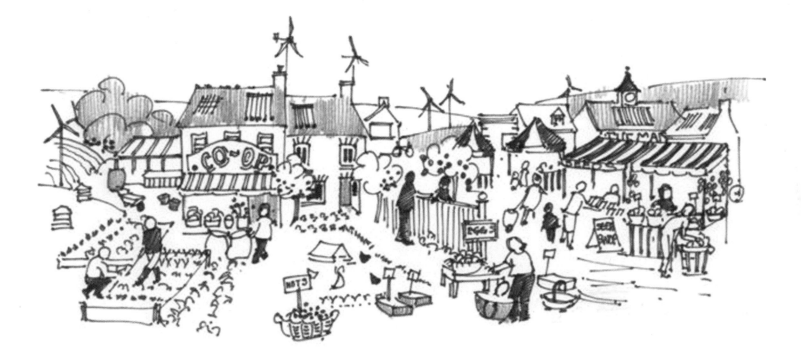

DEDICATIONS

To my mother, father and stepfather (without whom this book and my community would not be complete), my sister Ismay (who would have loved today) and my daughter Meli, who is the human embodiment of resilience and who this brighter, kinder world is for.

To Rob and Emma for their big-hearted support, constant inspiration, and their ability to make the most amazing of visions come true.

To Amanda and Alethea at Green Books for their warm patience and encouragement.

To the many, many people out there passionately contributing to a local food movement that feeds and nourishes hearts, bellies, minds, worms, birds, bees, skies and trees.

And to everyone who is and will be participating in the transition to community resilience, and who believes and demonstrates that change is possible, necessary and fun.

ACKNOWLEDGEMENTS

Many thanks to everyone who shared their words and stories with the readers of this book, including Teresa Anderson, Peter Andrews, Richard Arkwright, Tim Baines, Eva Bakkeslett, Jade Bashford, Dan Zev Benn, Joel Brook, Julie Brown, Lou Brown, Michael Brownlee, Rikke Bruntse-Dahl, Graham Burnett, Margaret Campbell, Jorge Carrion, Sue Clifford, Ingrid Crawford, Martin Crawford, Ann-Marie Culhane, Kath Dalmeny, Amanda Daniels, Clare Davies, Mike Downham, Fergus Drennan, Matt Dunwell, Hugh Fearnley-Whittingstall, Keith Goverd, Frank Hemming, Patrick Holden, Sue Holmes, Grifen Hope, Tom and Caz Ingall, Bob Jones, Sandor Katz, Ruth Kelly, Nick Kiddey, Eleanor King, Duncan Law, Caroline Lewis, Sheila Macbeth, Noni Mackenzie, Josiah Meldrum, Ross Menzies, Lisa Michael, Claire Milne, Abi Murray, Emma Noble, Alissa Pemberton, Julia Ponsonby, Kerry Rankine, Holly Regan-Jones, Richard Reynolds, Andrew Rundle-Keswick, Pete Russell, Eva Schonveld, Polly Senter, Kathryn Siveyer, Penny Skerrett, James Spriggs, Bethan Stagg, Kate Swatridge, Mark Thurstain-Goodwin, Susan Tivari, Robert Waldrop, Sue Walker, Jane Warring, Nick Weir, Claire White, Patrick Whitefield, Emma Winfield and Jonny Wood.

To the volunteer researchers who gave their time and expertise in the quest for local food stories and knowledge, including Josiah Meldrum, Alissa Pemberton, Kristin Sponsler and Beth Tilston, and a special big thank you to Hannah Roberson for her last-minute assistance with the finishing touches.

And to all the people, organisations and groups who have kindly shared images and illustrations, including Tom Beard, Canalside Community Food CSA, Common Ground, Ingrid Crawford, Fergus Drennan, Eastwood Comprehensive, Escoescuela El Manzano, The Former LETS allotment, Food Train, Geofutures, Growing Communities, Diane Lutzke, Graham Morgan photography, Pete Russell, Scott Morrison photography, Soil Association, St Ann's Allotments, Stroud Community Agriculture (SCA), Sustain, Sustainable Bungay, Sustaining Dunbar, Beth Tilston, Transition City Allotment, Transition City Canterbury, Transition City Nottingham, Transition Forest Row, Transition Town Glastonbury, Transition Town Kapiti, Transition Town Kinsale, Transition Town Lewes, Transition Town Totnes, Transition Town Tynedale, Transition Town West Kirby and Transition Town Westcliff.

FOREWORD

I've been in my role as the London Mayor's food advisor since the autumn of 2008, and on a daily basis I am astonished at how much exciting work is happening at the grassroots level – both in terms of food growing and of people seeking to lead a more sustainable lifestyle. Finally, it seems, we're truly waking up to what a strange world we have created for ourselves – one where job titles and fat salaries count for more than communities, and cheap, processed food has taken the place of locally grown, healthy and seasonable fare. It has come at a hideous price: the banking meltdown, an obesity and health crisis, and the fracturing of the ties that bind groups of people, which supply an essential sense of security and belonging.

The first Transition event I attended was in Lampeter, Wales, where 500 people rolled up to listen to Rob Hopkins talk about the Transition movement.* What was abundantly clear was that people wanted change and wanted to do anything to bring it about. Dig up the car park? Yes! Plant a garden in a local school? Yes!

We have become so disconnected from where our food comes from that many of us believe it just rolls off some conveyor belt in much the same way as nuts and bolts. But food is our primary need, and when we can reconnect children to the wonder of growing, the results can be astonishing. A National Farmers' Union survey undertaken as part of The Year of Food and Farming found that 93 per cent of primary-aged children who are exposed to growing their own food start to change their eating habits. It follows that the same is true for adults engaging in the kind of community food projects outlined in these pages.

It is thrilling for me to see our own Capital Growth initiative take hold in London. It is a simple scheme where groups of individuals who want to grow vegetables find spaces and then sign up to a growing group of like-minded people. All of the projects are community based and all of them help to provide the social cohesion that has been so lacking in our culture in the last three decades of 'me-me-me' thinking. As in this book, we tell people how to get started, but *Local Food* goes much further, giving you stories from the field as well as tips and resources for creating a range of food projects, from community allotments to farmers' markets. It is a serious hands-on guide that can empower us all towards local self-sufficiency and sustainability of our food systems.

I, like the vast majority, once thought that oil was an inexhaustible commodity. Now I know it's not – and, horrifyingly, in my lifetime, we've used up half of the world's supply. But perhaps peak oil couldn't have come at a better time: greenhouse gas levels are rising, our planet is in peril and it is up to all of us to endeavour to leave the world in good shape for following generations. This book is a very, very good place to start.

Rosie Boycott, May 2009

* See page 14 for information about the Transition movement.

INTRODUCTION

by Rob Hopkins

Echoes of a more resilient past

Not only is our entire agricultural and food system based upon the availability of cheap fossil fuels – we do not even use them in a wise and frugal manner. We squander them on flagrant consumerism in order to maximise short-term profit, while destroying the localised systems that once sustained our culture.

Dale Allen Pfeiffer

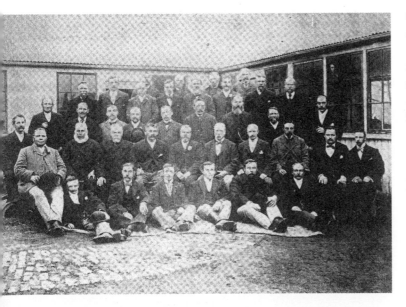

The photo on the left is one of my favourites. Taken in 1897, it shows the annual meeting of the Bristol and District Market Gardeners Association – thirty-seven men, in their Sunday best, posing for a formal photograph somewhere in Bristol. They sport a fantastic diversity of facial hair, and appear as smart, respectable members of the society of the time. Between them they managed many market gardens in and around the city of Bristol, creating livelihoods as well as a much more diverse and productive landscape than the one we see around us now. Today, no doubt, the sites where once they worked are host to car parks and concrete, rather than carrots and cabbages.

The steady and relentless erosion of the idea that food is something that grows near where you live, by someone you have some kind of a relationship with, and that you actually cook yourself, began after the Second World War and accelerated during the 1960s and 1970s. New subsidies and international trade agreements, accompanied by the rise of the super-market and the dazzling idea that you could now have whatever food you wanted from anywhere in the world, meant that it became, perversely, cheaper and easier to buy food grown many hundreds of miles away than food grown up the road. Farmers and growers went out of business with their land absorbed into larger farms. Orchards were grubbed out, our lives became saturated with processed foods and our waistlines started to bulge. The illusion of plenty came at a cost, as we discarded into the recycling bin of history a complex, highly skilled, adaptable and place-specific system that could be dismantled in a day but would take far, far longer to rebuild once it had gone.

Food security or food vulnerability?

During the 1930s, Britain's national food self-sufficiency declined precipitously, leaving it very vulnerable by the time of the outbreak of WWII. This led to a hastily introduced effort to build food security, with a combination of the Dig for Victory campaign and a huge increase in agricultural productivity (still seen by some as the heyday of British farming). Places that hadn't been dug or ploughed disappeared under productive use: Hampstead Heath, the flowerbeds around Buckingham Palace, and meadows and pastures were all rapidly pulled in to the national effort to avoid starvation. By the end of the war, 10 per cent of the nation's diet was coming from allotments and back gardens, and agricultural input had increased greatly. Nutritionists argue that the nation had never been healthier.

In the intervening years, national food self-sufficiency has ebbed and flowed, reaching a pinnacle in the 1980s. For a nation with such a rich history of fruit breeding, with many thousands of apple varieties suited to most soil types and climates, this is deeply perplexing, as well as troubling. If ever a country were ripe for a nationwide orchard-planting revolution, it is ours, and rediscovering the extraordinary diversity of our indigenous apples and the rich culture of songs, recipes, stories and festivals associated with them would be as much of a benefit as the rebuilding of our food security. Reacquainting ourselves with the Michaelmas Red, the Golden Noble, the Ribston Pippin, Ellison's Orange and the Pitmaston Pineapple would root us deeper in place, in culture and in history.

This erosion of our diverse, durable and resilient food system has all happened in the blink of an eye. Oral history interviews I have done in the South Hams in Devon describe how in the 1950s most houses had a vegetable garden; about a third of them kept chickens in urban back gardens; all meals were prepared using fresh ingredients; milk, fruit, meat and other foods were delivered to the home by local farmers and tradespeople; and the large majority of food consumed came from the local region – not out of some collective ethical choosing but through sheer practicality. Why import an apple from New Zealand when there are perfectly good ones growing a mile up the road? While this system wasn't perfect, it was a system of 'food feet' rather than 'food miles', and it worked. Although few today would tolerate an abattoir on their High Street, there is much about the idea of local food culture that we need to redesign for a modern context; the benefits of so doing would be legion.

Defra views any talk of food security as absurd. When it uses the word 'resilience' in the context of food, it is not talking about increased national production, about local markets and so on; rather it is talking about making the range of places the country sources its food from as diverse as possible. The broader the base, it argues, the less risk of any significant disruption to supply. Getting bananas from eight countries rather than four means we are less at risk. However, this attitude has started to shift. A recent Cabinet Office discussion paper on food security concluded that, in light of the challenge posed by climate change, "existing patterns of food production are not fit for a low-carbon, more resource-constrained future".[1] This book attempts to set out what 'patterns of food that *are* fit for a low-carbon, more resource-constrained future' might actually look like – and, indeed, are already looking like.

Why change is inevitable

Three factors are converging on our current models for how we feed ourselves, and they are converging very, very fast. The first is the issue of peak oil. In essence, oil is a finite resource, yet we continue to use it with reckless confidence, based on the assumption that we will always have it, in abundant supply and at reasonable cost. We have built infrastructure, living patterns and economic models on the understanding that we will always have access to this amazing resource, yet increasingly its uninterrupted supply is looking very vulnerable. We now consume four barrels of oil for each new one we discover, and more and more oil-producing nations are passing their peak of production.

The core of the peak oil issue is the following observation: that during what we might call The Age of Cheap Oil (from 1859 to the present), our degree of economic success and sense of personal well-being and prowess has been directly linked to our level of oil consumption, yet we are rapidly moving into a time where our degree of dependence equates to our degree of vulnerability. That is as much the case in terms of our food system as it is with anything else.

Secondly, the climate change issue means that the UK needs to begin driving its emissions down with an unprecedented sense of urgency. The most recent science on climate change shows that the world has reached some of the 'tipping points' predicted by climate scientists. Indeed, James Hansen of NASA has stated that the tipping point for the world's climate was actually 350ppm (atmospheric concentration of carbon dioxide, by volume, in parts per million)[2] – the fact that we are now at 387ppm being no reason why 350ppm should not remain the target. The important question is what the world would look like if we went to bed at the end of a day having sequestered (i.e. locked up in some way) more carbon than we emitted during that day. Some of the food strategies we will explore here are a part of that discussion. Making food and farming 'carbon positive' would mean that it would be *at the very least* organic (emissions from the use of nitrogen fertilisers are huge and are entirely unnecessary), as well as being more local, featuring more perennial crops such as productive trees, and, inevitably, employing more people.

The last factor is the economic contraction the world is presently experiencing, popularly known as 'the credit crunch'. The whole idea of perpetual growth was, if we're honest, absurd to start with. If we gauge the success or otherwise of our economies on whether year on year we consume more, buy more stuff and spend more money, we pretty soon hit up against the reality that the world is a finite resource, that there is no such place as 'away'. The economic recession we are going through now differs from previous recessions in that it is the first one under-pinned by an energy peak. Economic growth was made possible by a model that assumed that next year we would have more productivity, more cheap energy and therefore more economic activity than this year. With the growing acknowledgement that the age of cheap energy is behind us, the concept of growth is now looking increasingly absurd. And growth has come at huge cost – social, environmental and personal. A recent study showed that the last year that increased consumption made us any happier was 1961.[3] The sooner we are able to start designing for more realistic expectations of the future the better, as a more localised, diverse food system can't be cobbled together overnight: it takes design, forethought, money and a lot of work.

The role of Transition

The Transition movement (see www.transitionnetwork. org for more information) seeks to inspire, catalyse and support community responses to peak oil and climate change. Transition initiatives are intended to be a positive and solutions-focused response to the three interlinked challenges outlined on page 13. This is a process that acts as a catalyst for communities to begin an exploration of what life beyond cheap oil might be like, and then to design how, most effectively, they might begin preparing for it. It is positive, fun and engaging. From awareness-raising and forming local food groups to creating local currencies and developing 'Plan Bs' for their communities, those involved in the Transition movement seek to embrace the end of the Oil Age as being a tremendous opportunity – the opportunity for a profound rethink of much that we have come to take for granted. At the time of writing there are over 180 formal Transition initiatives, and thousands at earlier stages of the process.

There are Transition initiatives in the US, Japan, New Zealand, Sweden, Holland, Australia and many more besides. You will find them in towns and cities, on islands and in villages. There are now two local authorities (Somerset and Leicestershire) that have formally dedicated themselves to supporting these initiatives as they emerge. 'Transition training' has been set up to support these initiatives, and the training has been run around the world. There is a Transition consultancy, to work with businesses to look at how they can embed the idea of resilience in their work. Ambridge, in the fictional BBC Radio series *The Archers*, is a Transition Village. Ed Miliband, the Minister for Energy and Climate Change, recently told the Environment Agency conference in London that Transition initiatives were "absolutely essential". One of the first areas that Transition initiatives explore is that of food, as it is one of the issues people are most immediately interested in, and where there are many projects that can be started relatively quickly.

Two important caveats

This book does not, for a moment, argue that Transition initiatives are all we will need. Any successful navigation of the next twenty years will require action at international, national, regional and local levels, and at that local level will require a huge range of diverse organisations, many of which are signposted in this book. This diversity of organisations is what Paul Hawken describes in *Blessed Unrest* as the Earth's immune system kicking in, and this book celebrates that diversity rather than in any sense promoting Transition as a universal cure-all.

Secondly, the 'Cheerful Disclaimer' is that no one yet knows whether Transition will work. It evolves through constant iteration: people in communities on a range of scales try out the Transition process and then their experiences feed into the ongoing revision of the model. I think of it as one of the most important social research projects underway anywhere in the world. This book is, as much as anything, an invitation to be a part of the timely, urgent and historic process of designing a positive path through the near future, particularly in relation to food, whether you choose to call it Transition or not.

What food and farming need to be in the future

Given the need for an urgent and far-reaching rethink of everything we do, including how we feed ourselves, this may be an opportune moment to try to set out some kind of a vision as to what food and farming beyond the energy peak might be like. If we were to be able to taste, smell, hear and feel the UK in 2030, in relation to how it now feeds itself, what might it be like?

It would, out of necessity, be more focused on local markets, a low emitter of greenhouse gases, a user of far less water, free of its dependence on artificial fertilisers and chemical pesticides, a supplier of much more than just food (building materials, medicines and energy, for example), a far greater employer of people, and supported by a complex web of local processors and retailers. The rural landscape would not look exactly as it looks now; it would be far more diverse, home to a variety of land uses, with more tree cover and with less livestock. Soil building would have become a national obsession, given the powerful role that soils play in locking up carbon and the emissions that result from their neglect.

I would define the principles that will underpin this post-carbon way of feeding the country as follows.

- An approach that will play its full role in achieving the UK government target of an 80-per-cent cut in carbon emissions by 2050.
- Resilience, the ability at all levels to withstand shock, must be a key concept – embodied in the ability of the settlement in question, and its food-supply system, to adapt rapidly to rising energy costs and climate change.
- Improved access to nutritious and affordable food.
- Far more diversity than at present, in terms of species, ecosystems, produce and occupations.
- Prioritisation of the establishment of substantial carbon sinks through agriculture, so that farming is based more on perennial, tree-based systems, as well as good soil management and the return to soils of organic matter.
- More intrinsic links made to local markets than at present, with local produce being given preference wherever possible.
- A planned phase-out of dependence on fertilisers and other agrochemicals (ideally enabled by a shift to organic practices).
- A large increase in the amount of food produced from back gardens, allotments and more 'urban' food sources.
- No place for the use of genetically modified crops in what will be a more sustainable system of agriculture.

All of this leads to the question 'Can Britain feed itself?' Incredibly, this question has rarely been asked. In 1975 Kenneth Mellanby wrote a seminal study of that title,[4] which concluded that yes, the UK could still feed itself, but only if it ate a diet similar to that consumed in WWII, with the key determinant of success being the amount of meat produced. If, he argued, we ate meat like we did in 1945, i.e. a roast on Sunday, made into sandwiches on Monday, a soup on

FOOD ZONES: 80% SELF-SUFFICIENCY, 20% IMPORTS

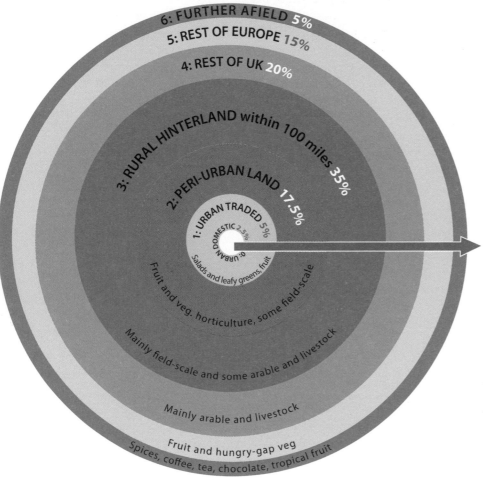

6: FURTHER AFIELD 5%
5: REST OF EUROPE 15%
4: REST OF UK 20%
3: RURAL HINTERLAND within 100 miles 35%
2: PERI-URBAN LAND 17.5%
1: URBAN TRADED 5%
0: URBAN DOMESTIC 2.5%

Salads and leafy greens, fruit
Fruit and veg. horticulture, some field-scale
Mainly field-scale and some arable and livestock
Mainly arable and livestock
Fruit and hungry-gap veg
Spices, coffee, tea, chocolate, tropical fruit

Moving from the inner to the outer rings we get:
• Decreasing perishability of produce
• Bigger plots available
• Increasing mechanisation
• Increasing carbon intensity of transport/distribution

As well as the distance from the urban centre, other factors that need to be taken into account in the choice of crops are the infrastructure and the soil type, topography and climate.

Grazing animals are included in the system where this makes sense. Pigs and chickens are fitted into mixed farming systems to use up waste and help improve soil fertility.

The urban population is gradually reduced as city dwellers move to the hinterland to get involved in farming and human labour becomes more significant.

Food zones, and the percentage of the total food supply sourced from each zone. This diagram is based on a model developed by Growing Communities in Hackney, London, showing what an urban-based, low-carbon, relocalised food system might look like in the future. The percentages given for each zone are based on Growing Communities' experience of setting up a local food system, and its achievements to date.

Tuesday and so on, we could still feed everyone from the UK's productive land.

Nobody asked the question again until 2008, when the editor of *The Land* magazine, Simon Fairlie, wrote an article by the same title – what he called 'a back of an A4 envelope' reappraisal of Mellanby's original study. [5] After looking at a range of scenarios, he concluded that the UK could still feed itself, and could do so organically, if, as Mellanby had also concluded, we eat less meat. He argued that there would also be sufficient space for growing more timber for fuel and construction as well as a range of other productive uses. While more research is needed here, and while total self-sufficiency is neither desirable nor possible, it is important to establish the level of self-reliance that is possible in order to start most effectively planning for its realisation.

One very useful model for how a future food system for this country might organise itself has been developed by Julie Brown of Growing Communities in Hackney, London. Growing Communities runs a number of food projects across its community, including a vegetable box scheme for over 450 people and a popular farmers' market (see Chapter 14 for a full description of its work). Based on the Growing Communities experience, Julie has developed what may well become the template for the food systems of the future – shown in the food zones diagram opposite. The model is a series of concentric rings, from the inner city in the middle to the rest of the world on the outer edge. Julie is starting to explore how replicable her model could be, both for urban and non-urban communities. In the context of this book, it is a highly useful model. In effect, this book focuses on the first three of Julie's rings, and on those initiatives that can be initiated by individuals and by community groups.

Ultimately, this is not just about farming, but rather about a move from a nation of farmers supplying a nation of passive consumers to a nation of producer-consumers, growing some of their own food, linked with local growers in a way that once again revalues food production as an art and a skill, and which treats food production on whatever scale with the esteem it lost some thirty or so years ago.

The place of this book in the local food movement

The idea of promoting local food production rather than relying unquestioningly on the globalised food system is not novel or in any way unique to this book. A rich and diverse web of allotment associations, farmers' markets, back-garden growers, food co-ops and seed swappers exists up and down the country, forming, for many years, the firm shoulders upon which this book, and the work of the myriad organisations promoting and implementing local food systems, stand. Many excellent organisations now actively promote local food, whether through growing, procurement or promotion (see the Resources section for full details).

A recent funding pot of £50 million called 'The Local Food Fund' has been specifically created in order to help drive this expansion forward.[6] City farms can be found in most cities, and even some artists have now begun seeing edible landscaping as an art form. Boris Johnson in London has initiated a programme to get 2012 food-producing gardens in place in time for the Olympics, and Blue Peter recently dug out its garden and put in vegetable beds. Manchester City Council is planning to spend £200,000 planting fruits, nuts and vegetables in every one of the city's parks.

This book sits in that context and performs two roles. Firstly, it is a celebration of the local food culture that already exists, and the extraordinary and dedicated people who have brought it into being and nurtured it over many years. Although much of the focus of this book is on what Transition initiatives are creating and catalysing, it is also very much placed in that wider context, and you will find a great deal of signposting to other related organisations and projects, as well as ideas for further research.

Secondly, this book is a handbook. It is intended to be a guide for anyone who would like to get a local food project off the ground and would like ideas and inspiration for practical projects. We hope that you will find it to be an inspiring and practical guide to get you under way in the most focused and effective way.

The wonder of reconnecting with food

I love my garden. Indeed, in many ways I am at my happiest in my garden. In my raised beds, built as terraces in my sloping garden, I grow carrots, beetroots, salads, spinach, chard, onions, kale, beans, peas and much more. Few things taste as good fresh from the garden as carrots and spinach. I don't grow food because I have to. It would, after all, be easier to buy it from the supermarket. I grow food because it feels fantastic to do so – it is a magical, almost alchemical, process that allows me to know what I am feeding my family, and that lets them connect what they eat with the beds they can see while they are eating it.

Similarly, the projects and initiatives set out in this book are not hair-shirt responses to impending catastrophe. They are the creation of people finding out that they share ideals and visions with each other,

and that they really enjoy working together to bring these visions to fruition. These are people who discover that growing some of their food is a learnable skill, not the metaphysical art they once believed it to be. They find that their kids become enthusiastic about food for the first time, and that they feel fitter and more connected to their community and to the soil. They are the desk-bound generation, living in an economy based largely, as the comedian David Mitchell recently observed, on 'ringtones and lattes', who discover the joys of planting out onion sets on sunny but chilly spring mornings. This is a book about people like you, who decide that they want to take back control of what they eat.

When food is once again central to our lives

It feels to me not only possible, but inevitable, that in ten years' time the Bristol and District Market Gardeners Association (and many others) will once again resume its annual meetings. The group will sit down together in a time when our views of the desirability of a career in growing food will have completely changed, and being an urban market gardener will be seen as a rather cool choice of occupation. These people will certainly not have quite such an extraordinary collection of facial hair, and there will be much more equal gender balance – indeed, if the proportion of people coming forward to take on allotments is anything to go by, the majority of them will be women.

Their occupation will be financially viable and deeply respected. They will be working in a very different world from today. The food footprint of our cities will have contracted considerably, and people's diets will be more seasonal. Their gardens will sit in a wider mosaic of productive back gardens, vibrant farmers' markets, fruit- and nut-tree plantings on city streets, school grounds reconceived as small farms, Community Supported Agriculture farms on the green belt land around the cities, and any free land that can be brought into productivity used for allotments and food gardens. It is my fervent hope that this book plays a vibrant role in bringing about this new food culture in as short a time as possible.

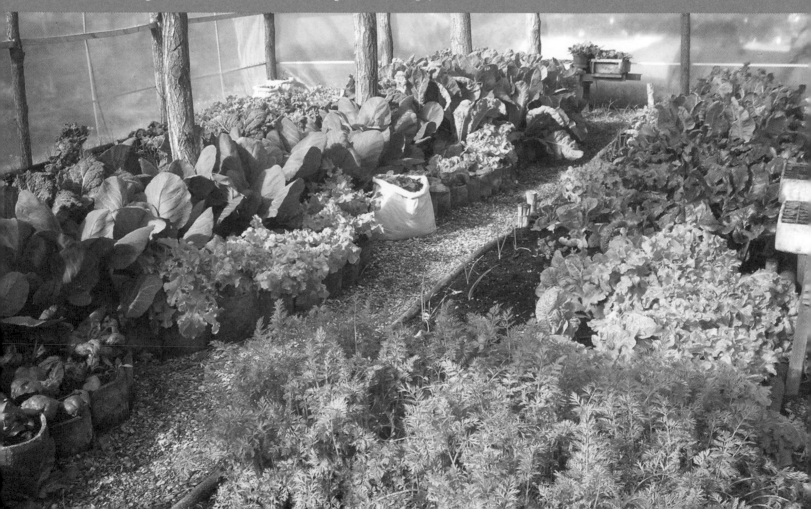

Productive local gardens will become a much more familiar sight in future. Photograph: Ecoescuela El Manzano

Chapter 1

THE LOCAL FOOD MOVEMENT

If fresh food is necessary to health in man and beast, then that food must be provided not only from our own soil but as near as possible to the sources of consumption. If this involves fewer imports and consequent repercussions on exports then it is industry that must be readjusted to the needs of food. If such readjustment involves the decentralisation of industry and the re-opening of local mills and slaughter-houses, then the health of the nation is more important than any large combine.

Lady Eve Balfour,
founder of the Soil Association, 1943

Given the degree to which the modern food system has become dependent on fossil fuels, many proposals for de-linking food and fossil fuels are likely to appear radical. However, efforts toward this end must be judged not by the degree to which they preserve the status quo, but by their likely ability to solve the fundamental challenge that will face us: the need to feed a global population of seven billion with a diminishing supply of fuels available to fertilise, plough, and irrigate fields and to harvest and transport crops.

Richard Heinberg
and Michael Bomford, 2009[1]

Food shapes and is shaped by many areas of our lives, from how we organise our days to the topography of our land, and much in between – our physical and emotional health; the climate; the quality of our air, water and soil; the diversity of the wildlife; the structure of our economies and the closeness of our communities. So it is perhaps not surprising that as change to the globalised, industrial food system is made inevitable by the limits of its own excesses (as discussed in the Introduction), one of the most popular focuses and starting points for many community-strengthening projects is the transformation and redefinition of the community's relationship to food – how it chooses to sow, grow, fertilise, harvest, sell, transport, source, buy, cook or eat it. In so doing, this process is helping to reinvigorate the local food networks, or 'foodsheds'[2] that once provided all of our food – webs of small-scale, commercial, non-profit-making and home-based producers, growers, processors and consumers, who are linked by face-to-face relationships and who share a local economy, environment and community.[3]

The shift towards local food is by no means happening only among the usual green suspects and the ranks of resource depletionists – it is also gathering momentum within the mainstream. This growing popularity has been reflected in recent research, with one UK study finding that 27 per cent of shoppers said they had bought local produce in the month prior to being surveyed, compared with 15 per cent three years ago.[4] Over in the US a similar shift is happening, with one in six American consumers recently questioned saying that they now go out of their way to buy local food as much as possible.[5] There does, however, seem to be a gap between this rise in demand for local food and what is currently being supplied. A further survey found that 70 per cent of UK consumers want to buy local and regional foods, but that 49 per cent would like to buy more than they do.[6] This last figure indicates that perhaps the amount and range of local food desired by consumers isn't always readily available or easily accessible, and that there are many gaps that the local food networks can fill with the shopper's blessing – or indeed, many potential converts to the art of small-scale food growing among the consumer masses. It may also indicate that the majority of shoppers are no longer content with the haze of blissful ignorance that glossy marketing and elongated supply chains perpetuate – a haze that has allowed the consequences of our buying habits to go largely unchecked for decades.

All the above figures suggest that a global economic slowdown does not necessarily imply a neglect of consumer ethics. Instead, the financial slump – accompanied as it is by the looming consequences of peak oil and climate change – has given us the opportunity to question the status quo and to realign our values with our lifestyles. The health of people and the environment, bound together by our need for food, is once again making its way up the priority list.

The welcome revival of local food in the UK, as well as in other countries around the world, is growing on the strength of years of groundwork carried out by communities and organisations in the field. Food Links UK, for example, was set up in 2002 as a network of organisations within the local food sector (including the Soil Association, Sustain, F3 and Food Matters), and has more recently merged with Sustain's Local Action on Food network. The network has been instrumental in establishing regional Food Links projects, such as Devon Food Links, East Anglia Food Links, and so on. The focus of each project has varied, but on the whole they have all facilitated a growth in local food networks in their areas by advising, funding, supporting and/or initiating local food projects, businesses, courses and events. One of the many Food Links success stories has been on the Isle of Skye in Scotland, which now boasts a Food Links van that delivers local produce to local businesses, a farmers' market, a community interest company and farmers' group dedicated to promoting local food and local food programmes in the island's schools (see www.tastelocal.co.uk to see the full range of their work). More recently, the Plunkett Foundation, together with a number of other local food organisations, has been allocated £10 million to roll out the Making Local Food work programme across the UK (see pages 165-9 for more on the mapping and community shop programmes it is engaged in, and www.makinglocalfoodwork.co.uk for full information).

But what exactly is local food? While we can define it in line with the principles laid out on page 15, it is up to the community projects working with local produce to determine the specifics of how far away their food is sourced, exactly what products are available within the established 'local' radius, how it is identified or verified, and how much or how little non-local produce it is acceptable to consume alongside it. Because the definition is dependent upon the context to which it applies, and because it is as locally specific as the produce it describes, there cannot be a one-size-fits-all set of defining criteria when it comes to local food. This is something that might frustrate any box-ticking or categorising efforts, but it is well suited to the creativity and community ingenuity typical of this food sector.

Throughout this book you will find groups coming up with their own definitions of local food that are tailored according to their visions of sustainable food production, the existence and range of specific projects and producers in the area, and the limits of resources and customer proclivity that determine the nature of each project's work. The food they call 'local' is sourced from anything between zero to over 150 miles away, and can be from within the same community, town, city, county or even region. Some food initiatives, such as Growing Communities in Hackney (page 159), or the Stroud Community Agriculture scheme (page 106) supplement their largely locally sourced produce with a small percentage of 'luxury' items from abroad, such as bananas and other shipped fruits (see the zones diagram on page 16 to find out what proportion of food Growing Communities sources from each zone). Others, like the Canalside Community Supported Agriculture scheme (CSA) (page 109) in Warwickshire, sell only their own-grown, seasonal produce to their members. But whatever their local food definitions currently are and whatever additional items they deal with alongside local produce, many of the projects we have looked at in the course of our research see themselves as being in the midst of a localising process, and hope to decrease the miles travelled by their produce as the local food movement grows and local food becomes easier to find.

From a consumer's point of view, it is important to point out that the local food movement isn't about denying British people the pleasures of sugar or coffee for ever more, nor about banning haggis for Londoners and Cornish pasties for the Welsh. Most local food supporters agree that a transition to greater food localisation doesn't mean imposing trade barriers and building walls of parochialism. Rather, it is about strengthening local food networks and shifting our focus back to home turf. That way, we can source most of our food from our immediate locality, while the food that is brought in beyond community, regional and national lines is done so as sustainably as the extended food miles will allow (i.e. with the same respect for producers, adherence to organic standards, and with as minimal a dependence on fossil fuels as possible). As the import-hungry developed world relocalises its tastes and purchases, this will also allow producers and farmers overseas to concentrate on feeding their own communities and nourishing their own soil, instead of working to satisfy the whims of fluctuating international food markets and the profit-chasing aims of multinational food businesses.[7]

The enjoyment of long-distance-traded, non-native foods is a luxury that future resource limitations may well halt, and British chocoholics will then have to be incredibly creative about how they satisfy their fix. But weaning ourselves off our favourite faraway foods is a process that won't happen in a day. Again, within the throngs of shoppers actively supporting local produce there is a spectrum of ideals being played out at the cash till, as the hard-line 'locavores' choose to eat within only a 30-mile radius of their home, while others permit themselves cups of tea, rice milk, bananas and Italian wines to accompany their garden-, orchard- and local-farm-sourced meals.

Beyond drawing the local food boundaries, projects featured in this book also have different standards when it comes to how the food they deal with is produced, focusing on what is organic and certified, organic and not certified, wild or biodynamic – or some combination of the above. There are also some projects that choose to prioritise local food over organics or vice versa. But, whatever side of the various food fences they fall on, they are all part of an evolving and highly varied movement around local food that no one can typify.

This book focuses predominantly on the fruit and vegetable sector of local food, which reflects the make-up of the local food movement in its current state. But as local food networks become more sophisticated – as diets shift and infrastructure for local food production is developed – the growing of grains, nut trees and/or the keeping of livestock will have to feature more widely across our localised foodsheds if we are to remain well fed beyond the oil peak. And, as our communities are reskilled, more of us will be able to participate in the growing and rearing of plants and animals that can provide us with the protein and carbohydrates that we need – not to say the wine, honey and sugar that we also enjoy. So, in perhaps twenty years' time, a new edition of this book might have chapters dedicated to community nut plantations, bee-keeping co-ops, community dairies and community grain stores, together with a particularly dense chapter on community vineyards and breweries. In the meantime, there are many people across the globe today who are experienced and engaged in small or polycultural large-scale nut and grain growing or livestock keeping, and their knowledge can help to expand the focus of the local food movement in the years ahead.

As with the intertwined issues of climate change, peak oil and economic meltdown, it is unhelpful (and potentially dangerous) to dissect and isolate any of the motivations and principles that guide, or the links that comprise, local food networks. If we do, valuable and vital elements of these food systems could be lost along the way. Local food networks are not, for example, simply about reducing the amount of carbon in the food chain. A focus on CO_2 emissions belies the fact that the majority of the UK's agricultural greenhouse gas emissions are from methane and nitrous oxide (the latter, mainly sourced from artificial fertilisers, being 310 times more damaging than CO_2).[8] A focus on carbon reduction as the solution to more sustainable food production also says very little about how a community might become empowered to determine its own food supply, to eat more nutritious foods, or to communicate with the people that grow it. At the same time, an economics-based assessment of local food (while research proves that a local food economy makes financial sense[9]) ignores those elements of local food networks that cannot be counted, such as the strengthening of social relationships as food supply chains contract, or the deep appreciation of life in nature that comes with growing your own food. At the same time, a focus on organic produce can obfuscate the fact that while an organic mango may be a healthier fruit than a pesticide-sprayed apple, its transportation to the UK is polluting and its nutritional content compromised by the miles it covers.

The alternative model of food systems that the local food movement is building therefore needs to encompass every facet of a community's relationship to food, from establishing fair farmers' wages to ensuring that rivers run free of pollution; from limiting diet-related, life-threatening illnesses among humans to supporting local bird populations. If a transition in food is to be realised, it has to be thorough. Having said that, we are in the midst of a rapidly changing time and, as each community grapples with the transformations it wants to set in motion, priorities will vary, perspectives will clash, tastes will differ and balances will tip towards and away from sustainability as we try to find our fossil-fuel-free feet. But there is enough space within the principles of Transition and the local food movement generally to accommodate all of these shifts and fluctuations. As too is there space for a variety of food philosophies (including those held by vegans, vegetarians, raw-food enthusiasts, wild-food foragers and meat-eaters[10]), as well as a range of food-growing approaches (including organic,[11] biodynamic,[12] forest-gardening[13] and permaculture[14]-inspired food production), with all the disagreements and creativity that may arise between them. The people best placed to respond to the food issues that face us are those who make up the colourful, growing-to-eating spectrum within each local community as it forges its own path to resilience.

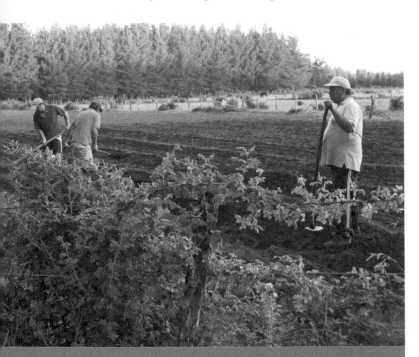

Out in the fields in Chile's first Transition group in El Manzano, Biobio. Photograph: Ecoescuela El Manzano

Using this book

As mentioned in the Introduction, the purpose of this book is to celebrate existing local food projects, and to provide inspiration, generate ideas and encourage community action around local food issues. The projects featured in these pages have been chosen because they are innovative, interesting and/or examples that others can learn from. Between them they make up a vibrant cross-section (but by no means an exhaustive list) of local food work that is happening in various communities across the Transition Network and beyond. Transition initiatives are relatively young newcomers to the local food scene, and, as we shall see, much of the food-related work that has grown up within them has been and will continue to be informed, influenced and inspired by the work of other projects.

This book is predominantly UK-based, but it includes a few examples of projects located elsewhere in the world, to give a sense of the relevance that a transformation in food also has in other cultures, and to show how far and wide the local food movement is spreading. The variety is broad – from one-off projects that require relatively little planning and funding through to long-term, larger-scale initiatives that entail ongoing dedication, money and time. The point here is partly that people and communities are as diverse as the actions that change them, but also that effecting change is possible at many different levels, from the small to the large, the short- to the long-term, the easy to the complex. From establishing a community garden to simply giving a spinach seedling to a neighbour, every act in the direction of greater food resilience is a valid, valuable part of the process of relocalisation. As the American activist Rebecca Solnit points out, ". . . history is shaped by the groundswells and common dreams that single acts and moments only represent . . . And though huge causes sometimes have little effect, tiny ones occasionally have huge consequences."[15] As we all know, the tiniest of seeds can produce the most magnificent of trees.

Community projects are, by their nature, often hard to squeeze into any one category because they evolve according to the idiosyncracies of their community and environment, and because they may change and expand their scope as their work develops. Many of them also prefer to resist being put in any kind of labelled box that might tighten their identity or dictate their path. So the categories that are used for the purpose of this book, and that form the titles for each chapter, are to be taken lightly – the projects within them aren't necessarily *only* community gardens, farmers' markets and so on; nor has each project interpreted the category titles in the same way. Moreover, it is possible that in the space of time between the research being conducted and you reading these pages, some of the featured projects could well have taken on an entirely new shape or direction beyond the category we have placed them in.

Within the following chapters there is some background information on the category itself, followed by stories of relevant projects and the people that run them. Towards the end of the book, Chapter 15 looks at 'Yet more inspired ideas' within the local food movement, with a brief description of other types of local food project that are worthy of attention.

We have presented the featured projects as stories rather than as a list of chronological bullet points, in order to give space to the unique shape and history of each project. Putting the projects into their own contexts in this way also emphasises that there is not one gardening glove that fits all when it comes to community work on local food, and that it is up to readers to draw their own conclusions, inspiration or lessons from each story rather than taking it as a blueprint for similar future action.

Project members who have written to us, or whom we have met or spoken with, have offered tips for others wanting to embark on similar work, and these are shown at the end of each chapter. There are also recommended websites, books, helpful organisations and relevant contacts to accompany each chapter, which can be found in the Resources section at the end of the book. In Chapter 16 there are suggested general steps for how to set up a local food project of your own, followed by ways of reaching out to other local food initiatives in your community and across the local food movement.

Many of the projects on these pages are small initiatives run by a few dedicated people using little resources but much of their own time. So we would kindly ask that you bear this in mind and be sensitive to the limits of their energy and workloads if you are considering sending them requests for assistance, opinions or guidance for your own projects. While some will be better placed to share their experiences more widely or to mentor, give talks or write articles, others may simply not be able to do so. A number of those featured have their own websites, so have a look through these first to see if they have the information you're looking for.

A transition in food

Patrick Holden

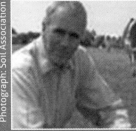

Photograph: Soil Association

I believe that Transition is an idea whose time has come and that it is no accident that millions of citizens all over the world have been inspired by the idea of taking direct action at a personal and community level to prepare for the future.

What is clear is that one of the first and most decisive actions that we can take in relation to the transition proposition is to change our relationship with our food, and this is where the Soil Association comes in.

To anyone who still questions the importance of food in the transition process I would say this – in relation to climate change and fossil-fuel depletion, there is likely to be a serious food crisis long before the effects of global warming impact on our lives. This will be caused by the accumulative consequences of a century of treating fossil-fuel energy, soil fertility, water and other 'earth capital' as if it were income. Dealing with the consequences of living beyond our means in this way will require the biggest change in our food and farming systems since the industrial revolution, and we have perhaps fifteen years at best to put in place the necessary changes to protect our food systems for future generations. One of the most important steps we can take as consumers is to buy local, organic food wherever possible, as this action alone supports the growers, producers and sellers that are working to put these changes in place. But as community members there is much more we can do besides, as this book demonstrates.

The Soil Association has a responsibility, as the national organisation promoting sustainable agriculture, to do everything we can to assist the Transition movement in shifting towards sustainable, local food systems, whether by assisting community groups to set up CSAs or transform their schools' food culture, or by collaborating on projects to reconnect producers and consumers. As a way of demonstrating our commitment to this cause, and to help establish strong links between the Transition movement and the Soil Association, I am personally committed to speak to Transition food groups on the subject of food and farming in transition whenever this is practically possible.

Patrick Holden is an organic farmer based in West Wales, and the Director of the Soil Association, the UK's leading organic certification body. The Soil Association is at the forefront of enabling and campaigning for a greater production of organic, local food (see www. soilassociation.org.uk).

Opening up the community space

One of the aims of community-based food projects is to open up the community space between individuals and the structures of government and business; to enable, show and remind people that they can determine their own worlds, build their own power and confidence, and significantly transform their food culture. If we assume that the only powers capable of effecting change are in the hands of government officials and corporate CEOs, then growing and sourcing local food for our families and communities may not seem like a radical, world-saving act. But if we grant ourselves the possibility that we can, at the home and community levels, transform the food systems around us, then every small step towards this transformation becomes relevant. And, if we are to tip the balance of national self-reliance back in our favour, we need all the growing help we can muster – each pair of hands being a crucial part of a large-collective effort. This doesn't mean that community interaction with local, regional and national government and business is not important and that the community is an island off the policy-making, deal-brokering main shore. The recent, and ongoing, work of pesticides campaigner Georgina Downs (in single-handedly securing a legal victory against the UK government for neglecting the safety of rural communities due to pesticides exposure – see www.pesticidescampaign.co.uk) is just one example of how an ordinary individual can respond to and change national legislation. Some of the groups described in this book have also been busy liaising and negotiating with businesses, and with local and national governmental bodies, as of course have the many food-focused national charities and non-profit-making organisations in this country and abroad. These efforts are a crucial part of the bigger local food picture, and it is important to remember that decisions made at the strategic and legislative levels have the potential to effect profound, positive change in each stage of the food supply chain, from the planting of a seed to the eating of a meal. But, while multilateral engagement and communication has its place, our main focus here is to revive *community* action around food; to encourage people from all places and backgrounds to look within themselves to find the solutions, energy and power necessary to stay healthy and fed for generations to come.

As this book is being written the local food movement is growing, evolving and taking on new shapes in the communities that nurture it. These communities that are reclaiming their right and ability to make change happen include villages, towns, cities, forests and islands – so, as we shall see, the range of projects emerging from them is just as varied. This book is therefore designed to appeal to community groups of whatever size, shape and location. It is also purposely non-prescriptive or directive, but is simply a tool, providing groups with inspiration and signposts to accompany the creativity, ideas and passion they already have. Steps and tips are suggestions for action that groups can mull over and use as they see fit, and are by no means the only way of doing things. The speed of evolution within the movement means that there are many ideas, models and edible epiphanies besides those listed here that will arise in the future (some perhaps springboarding from this very book). So, while we cannot describe or represent a destination in local food work, this book is instead part of a momentum that we hope to help nourish.

The definition of 'community group' used here is intentionally loose, to include all the forms such groups might take, but it refers essentially to a group of people who are connected through the place in which they live (anything from a rural hamlet to a city), and the resources, environment and society that they share. The community groups we look at in this context also share a passion for local food and a desire to make it more widely available. While not all projects featured evolved from the community sphere (some, for example, were initiated by national organisations), those that did not are here because of the validity of their work or the assistance that their programmes can offer community groups, or because community groups might find their models helpful.

Themes across local food projects

In researching community food projects, certain themes have emerged that are helpful in understanding the local food and Transition movements. The themes are not necessarily common to all community food projects (featured or not), but they point towards significant trends that may be of help in informing the newer initiatives yet to emerge.

Shared ownership

Within many of the projects looked at in this book there is a willingness and determination to share responsibility between all the members and to make every member feel as though he or she has an important part to play. This is so even when specific tasks have been assigned to each member, so that all tasks and roles are given equal worth. Some of the projects have shared ownership in place from the outset, whereas others come to it as they grow and more members are pulled in. In terms of how the projects interact with the world beyond their work, every food community project we encountered has been happy to share its ideas and experience with others, and some actively make their stories, tools and methods available for other groups wanting to do similar work. This is a radical move away from our legally sanctioned obsession with private ownership that can encourage suspicion and fear of what it might mean to share.

Shared decision-making

This theme is linked to that above, and refers to the way groups go about making decisions and organising roles within their project. For many community projects, this is an integral part of what they are about – creating a space in which involved community members can have a say in the project's direction and shape. In the projects we have looked at this has been manifested in different ways, so that some may have elected management groups in which decisions are made by consensus only, others may be run democratically across the whole group, and others still may have a leader who draws all other members' opinions and perspectives into the decision-making process. Opening this process up to wider debate can make it lengthy and sometimes incredibly difficult to arrive at a decision, but it is often worth the effort of balancing the power and sifting through the issues that define a project's work.

Moving beyond our comfort zones

It is inevitable that most people involved in food relocalisation will find themselves at some point being taken out of cheap-energy-furnished comfort zones and put into new roles that they find difficult, painful or just plain tedious. While this is now arguably a matter of choice, it will become unavoidable as resource depletion sets in. Departure from the comfort zone is a noticeable theme within local food projects that have already emerged, with many people giving up part of their work and income to have more time for home or community food projects, cutting down or eliminating 'luxury', non-local foods from their diets, or taking on labour-heavy skills and lifestyle changes instead of going for the 'easy' fossil-fuel option. If we start to do this now instead of waiting until transport systems and energy supplies collapse, we will be more prepared for times ahead – while hopefully finding ourselves creating alternative 'zones' that are not only more resilient but, once the shock of change has passed, more socially, economically and environmentally comfortable too.

Reconnection with place

A number of food-project participants have found that a focus on local produce through community-engaged action has reconnected them with the place in which they live, its nature and its seasons, so that it is now not only their home but also the source of their food and where new friendships and networks are nurtured. This revaluing of place and the people living and growing within it helps to put a 'face' back on the food produced, and trust back in the supply chain. It also brings local growers, sellers and buyers back in touch with the food traditions and recipes of their area, developed over generations to make best use of the food that their local land could provide.

Creativity

There is an astonishing amount of creativity in the types of local food project that are springing up, both in terms of what they are about and how they are being run. This is probably due in part to the above themes that cut across them and that help to encourage an open atmosphere where idea-conjuring and idea-moulding can thrive. But it is also about people following their passion for local food, and caring deeply about preserving and propagating the networks that support it – they are determined that their projects will succeed and they will go to great lengths to ensure they do. Some of the featured projects we encountered have chosen to protect their creativity through a constitution or set of principles, by not going for any external funding, or by bypassing or downplaying the role that money has in the project's development. Others actively encourage creativity within the group through regular visioning, brainstorming or mind-mapping exercises. However it is protected or encouraged, a respect for creativity will help projects to adapt to changes within and around them, and to make the most of any limitations or new territories they come across.

Building alternatives

> You can never change things by fighting the existing reality. To change something, build a new model that makes the existing model obsolete.
> Buckminster Fuller

Building positive, vibrant alternatives to the structures that depend on the perils of cheap energy is an integral part of what the Transition movement is about, and the same Fuller philosophy underpins many of the local food projects that have grown up within and beyond this movement. A number of the projects we looked at have explicitly chosen not to engage with systems and organisations they see as confounding the resource scarcities we face. This makes their job harder and can require an amazing amount of ingenuity and will (especially when much of the food world appears to be carrying on as though

Kenyan beans will be a staple part of the British diet for generations to come). But if relocalised food networks are to be realised, it is imperative that we have some projects out there that fully embody the oil-free vision and that prove to those of us in the oil-dependent present that it is indeed possible to dispense with the black gold and still have a full belly.

Sowing and reaping

This last theme is about how, by sowing ideas in the community sphere, many local food projects manage to meet their needs through connections and inter-actions with other community members. Many food-project participants have commented on how the resources, funds, materials and venues they needed were offered when asked for in the community – something that is often astounding in our culture where we are no longer accustomed to turning to the community for help. Some might put this down to serendipity, happy coincidence, good luck or sheer cheekiness on the part of some determined local

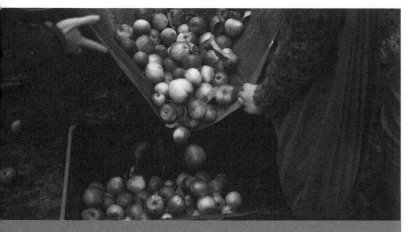

Juicing apples gleaned by Abundance project volunteers in Sheffield (described on page 169). Photograph: Anne-Marie Culhane

foodies, but, whatever you choose to call it, an ethically based, community-run local food project whose time has come is often a magnet for offers of assistance from the wider community. A cautionary note, however: we are not claiming that every community food project will always get what it wants by virtue of its good intentions and pester power, simply that it is certainly worth asking!

Seven principles for community-based local food projects

The following principles have been designed with Transition initiatives in mind,[16] but they can also be used by other community-based local food projects to help determine what kind of local food work their members might engage in, and how they might go about doing it (see Chapter 16 for more on how to set up a local food project).

1. Positive visioning

The process of visioning, of exploring in detail how group members would like their food project or even the wider local food movement to grow, can be a deeply powerful tool that helps to clarify and unify the group's intentions from the outset. This does not mean to say that individual visions within the group need to be synchronised in order for the project to work. In fact, differences between the visions of group members can be a useful source of debate and creativity. But the visioning process is important for opening up communication and for freeing visions – in all their commonalities and differences – that are held by the group. Once created, these visions can be used as touchstones to help navigate through unclear or tricky times. The creation of visions does not have to imply a clinging to what is conjured up. Rather, they are more powerful if held lightly and if they are responsive to the changes and unforeseen happenings that may occur as the project develops. Over time, it might therefore be necessary to re-vision, or to modify the original plan within the context of group cooperation.

However groups decide to go about visioning (whether it involves using paints, glue, potatoes or simple words[17]), it is important that each member has the opportunity to explore and share his or her vision in full. To accompany this process, it might help to research or visit food projects doing similar work, or to spend some time volunteering with them. Positive visioning could even be turned into a community-wide exercise, with other local food projects, Transition initiative food groups or interested members of the public being drawn into the process. Shaun Chamberlin's book *The Transition Timeline* can be a useful tool to help set the future, post-cheap-energy stage for visioning work.

2. Help people access good information and help them to make good decisions

This principle refers to the way Transition initiatives present and enable access of information around the issues they have emerged to tackle, and it is equally relevant for local food projects in general. Each project has a responsibility to enthuse, engage and 'impassion' its members and the public to work towards greater, community-embedded food resilience. This means encouraging awareness around the issues they address with accurate, clear descriptions of their principles and the data and arguments that support them – through leaflets, websites, public presentations or whatever medium they choose to use. But it is up to each person, project and initiative to draw their own conclusions and determine their own directions based on this

sound evidence, and part of sharing this information is trusting that those you share it with will make good, ethically responsible local food decisions that will serve the local food network as a whole.

3. Inclusion and openness

The fundamental need for food is something that crosses all social and political boundaries, and that can draw together the most diverse mixes of people. It is therefore a particularly effective focus area when working to achieve inclusion in a community. As mentioned earlier, sourcing wholesome, local, organic food is no longer seen as being the exclusive domain of 'green' people – instead, a spreading concern for human and environmental health is convincing more of us that access to such food is a right held by all, and a fundamental element of any sustainable, resilient community.

Community food projects are springing up in the grounds of inner-city estates as well as in the gardens of wealthy market towns. Even those projects that are located on one site (as opposed to being mobile or made up of a number of plots) can provide opportunities to bring people together by drawing in volunteers from various backgrounds in the surrounding areas. Some creativity may be required to bring inclusion about, but the project (and the reach of its message) will benefit as a result. Transparency of the project's aims, activities and expenditure can help to project an air of honesty, attract a wider audience to its work and inspire trust amongst local residents that engage with it. When a project opens its gates and doors to all sectors of its community, its message goes further, its resource pool is wider, and its support network is stronger.

A move towards greater community inclusion and openness is crucial in this era of peak oil, climate change and economic contraction, as we can no longer afford to languish in the comfort of 'sticking to our own'. A straddling of the divisions between us is part of rising to the challenges we face, not only because we need all available hands, but also because these challenges will affect all of us irrespective of socio-economic status or political and moral values. Well-off suburbanites in the Surrey green belt will be as vulnerable to food insecurities as factory workers living in downtown Sheffield, if both groups put no plans in place to grow, produce and source food in their local areas. A transformation in food culture needs to happen everywhere and with society-wide support.

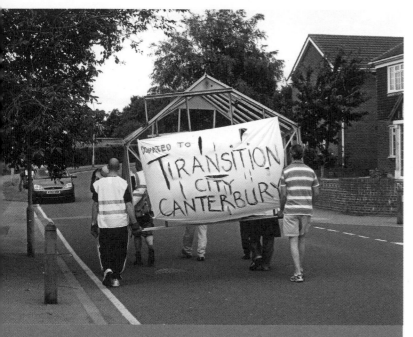

The Transition City Allotment team in Canterbury carrying the Transition Network's biggest sandwich board to their plot (with a newly donated greenhouse to go with it).
Photograph: Transition City Allotment

4. Enable sharing and networking

Some food projects, especially those that have a visible presence in the community, promote awareness of local food issues simply through their existence – people notice and take interest in what they're doing, and popularity is spread through word of mouth. But by communicating the project's aims and principles alongside its work (in the form of leaflets, noticeboards, banners, open days, etc.), a community group can make its vision go further. Whether promotion is about recruiting more voluntary workers or encouraging members of the public to visit or support the project, it is always an opportunity to spread awareness about the local food movement at large and the motivations for it. To do this in a way that is clear, accessible and entertaining means that the message will be received and understood by more people, and that it is more likely to be picked up by local and national media. This approach will also help to address the challenge of reaching the unusual suspects – of putting ideas of food resilience on the radar of people who are yet to learn about peak oil and the consequences it will have for the contents of our kitchen cupboards. This kind of promotion could be done from the beginning, or further down the line once more time and resources become available.[18]

It is also crucial that individual projects within the local food movement share, document, discuss and publicise their experiences and learnings (the good, the bad and the ugly), so that others can benefit from their efforts. See pages 179-83 for ways of establishing communication channels between local food initiatives and across the networks they are a part of.

5. Build resilience

The concept of resilience[19] is crucial at all levels of food culture change, from small-scale community food projects through to global efforts to relocalise food production and minimise unnecessary trade. As the focus here is on the community level, resilience can be used to guide not only 'what' a food project is working to achieve (an ongoing supply of safe and nutritious food in the post-fossil-fuel era) but also 'how' it is being carried out.

Based on what we know from the discipline of ecology, there are three ways in which an ecosystem, or in this case a community food initiative, can build resilience. Firstly, a project can draw strength from fostering diversity in terms of the backgrounds of project members, the skills they have and the sources of advice and information that are used. On the ground level, it is also important to promote diversity in the planning and growing of crops (so as to encourage good soil quality, flourishing wildlife and protection against the failures or diseases of particular crops). Promoting diversity in all areas of the project's work will help to ensure its flexibility and ability to withstand unforeseen changes and events. The project will contribute more to the resilience of a community if it is part of a diverse local food system – one that is made up of a variety of schemes such as community orchards, Community Supported Agriculture schemes (CSAs), garden share schemes and food cooperatives.

A second aspect of a food project's resilience relates to how it is organised. There is no one model that all projects should follow, and those featured here have found their own place that suits them on a spectrum between formality and informality. But if there is group agreement from the outset on how the project will be structured (whether this is achieved through consensus or democratic process), there is a much higher chance that it will run efficiently and with minimal misunderstandings between members – even if it is intended to be as formless and bureaucracy-free

as possible. A central principle of organising for resilience is to work towards group cooperation and mutual respect, which for many necessitates taking a flat-structured, non-hierarchical approach. At the same time, striking a balance between the independence and cooperation of group members means that the project as a whole can function in the absence of one of the team, and also that any one member is able to carry out his or her role without complete reliance on the rest of the group.

Lastly, how a group communicates is a crucial part of its resilience, both internally and with the wider local food system that it is part of. For the project itself this is partly down to a matter of scale (of ensuring that it does not grow to the point where efficiency or good communication might be compromised), but it is also about making sure that rules and principles are developed and understood between project members, and that there are regular opportunities for issues to be aired and relationships to be strengthened. The project will benefit from staying in close communication with other local food initiatives and, if relevant, the wider Transition group in its area; sharing knowledge, information and news, and perhaps tools, venues, processing facilities and labour too.

6. Inner and outer Transition

An integral part of the Transition approach is to encourage engagement with the movement through the promotion of positive visions (as described on pages 30-31), the creation of safe spaces to explore relevant issues and generate ideas, and the affirmation and celebration of work that is carried out. Behind this is an awareness that a shared sense of empowerment and passion grows more effectively in a nurturing, trusting and happy environment, rather than in one steeped in suspicion and fear of what might come.

This is as true for a small allotment project as it is for a Transition initiative or a community as a whole.

There is also something here about the importance of withholding judgement on others. Within the local food movement there is a wide spectrum of participants – some who choose not to own cars, some who fly, some who shop at supermarkets and some who only eat locally. To cast judgement on people and on behaviour that falls short of localist 'ideals' only contributes to guilt, communication breakdown and, crucially, inaction. Each person needs to be able to determine his or her own 'ideal' and work towards it without the fear of being criticised by others who are further down the path. In short, we need to be respectful of each individual's rate and shape of their own inner and outer transition, and what they choose to prioritise within that process.

This accepting, but positively proactive, approach is reflected in the work of many community food projects. Rather than urging people to protest 'against', and be judgemental of the structures that delocalise our food, they are enabling communities to be 'for' food resilience and to help create alternatives that work well. This empowering 'call to spades' is about devising abundant, beautiful, fun and delicious food projects that others want to be a part of, and about reaching the collective mind through the collective eyes, heart, hands and belly.

7. Subsidiarity: self-organisation and decision-making at the appropriate level

The food projects that follow are testament to the ability of community groups to self-organise, make decisions that mitigate the effects of food insecurity and inspire local food networks to grow. These projects are opening up the space between action on the scale of the individual home-garden grower and that of national agricultural policies – and it is a space in which much can be done and change can occur. The more that communities draw together around food and rediscover their own abilities to shape the foodscapes around them, the more the benefits of cooperative action will be seen, valued and acted upon by other neighbours and policy makers across the country and beyond. We have everything we need to build food resilience in our communities and it is up to each of us to help make it happen.

Resources

See page 203 for Local food – general.

Chapter 2

THE GREAT RESKILLING

The massive environmental and social changes that we face will affect not only how we produce, harvest, share and sell our food but also what we eat and how we eat it. If communities are to reclaim food production and supply chains from the environmentally damaging and nutritionally reckless systems of today, people within them need to be reskilled – that is, we need to relearn all the skills and trades that once made up the thriving local food economies of a pre-oil society and that will help us to steer a steady course through the times of unprecedented change that lie ahead.

The Great Reskilling process is step 8 of setting up a Transition initiative (see *The Transition Handbook* for more details) and is an integral part of any community's transition to a more resilient future. Beginning with one-off workshops, talks and courses, this process might eventually lead to reskilling schools popping up across the world, offering training in bread making, sauerkraut production and composting. But wherever this reskilling path might take us, we can start to think now about what skills we will need individually and pooled within a community in order to support a successful local food network.

Have a quick look around your kitchen and pick out food items that have arrived there with the help of fossil fuels – whether through fertiliser, herbicide or pesticide use, transportation or packaging – and think about what skills (and materials) might be necessary to help stock your cupboards with similar or replace-ment products once cheap energy dwindles. Growing your own is an obvious part of solving the post-peak-oil food dilemma, but there are many other skills that we can explore, such as preserving foods for winter, collecting, storing and saving seeds, baking breads, cooking without fossil fuels or identifying, preparing and eating wild local plants. The skills each of us choose to acquire will of course depend upon our individual and community tastes and needs. Having community facilities such as a local bakery, abattoir or juice press will also help to reduce the reskilling burden placed on individuals within that community.

There are two ways of going about reskilling for food security – either under the tutelage of an experienced person already skilled in his or her art, or, if such a person isn't readily available, embarking on the learning process unguided (alone or as part of a group of other keen reskillers). Transition Town Kapiti's Travelling Garden Group (see page 76) is one good, group-based example of the latter, where participants share, reskill and learn together. The former provides a way of valuing the skills and wisdom of those who know how to make the fossil-fuel-free eating experience not only possible but also fun, nutritious and delicious. Many such people can be found within the ranks of a community's older generation, which grew up in a time when cheap oil was yet to seep into every aspect of human society. Asking them to help reskill a new generation of oil-free growers and cooks is a way of bridging gaps between the young and the old, and of reconnecting younger community members with the history and culture of the place in which they live. But there is also a growing swell of knowledgeable and experienced teachers from younger generations who are happy and willing to share their passion with community groups keen to learn more. Check out some of the course centres on page 194, local food organisations on pages 203-5 and Great Reskilling resources on page 201-2 to track down relevant teachers.

Many Transition initiatives worldwide (including those in Hereford, Kilkenny, Lewes and beyond) have organised projects, workshops, courses and events to provide locals with the skills and understanding they need to grow their own food. And many experienced teachers who are part of these initiatives have instigated their own community projects to help support local food-security efforts. The following are two examples of 'Great Reskilling' projects run by Transition initiatives, together with articles by respected food lovers and teachers, which might help to inspire creative thinking and ideas around food reskilling.

Great Reskilling stories

Project name: The No-Dig Gardening Project

Location: Nelson, South Island, New Zealand

Aim: To train local people in a no-dig approach to food production, and to encourage community engagement with local food.

Started: 2008

How many people involved: One teacher, fifteen workshop participants.

On the web: www.transitionnelson.org.nz/no-dig-workshops

The idea

As mentioned earlier, 'how to grow' workshops and courses have been converting local residents to the way of food growing in a number of Transition initiatives. One such project is found in the New Zealand city of Nelson, on South Island. Bob Jones, an experienced gardener now living in the area, originally helped establish the organisation Grow Food Not Lawns in Colorado, USA in 2007. Now working with the Transition City Nelson folk, he has initiated a similar project there – the No-Dig Gardening Project – which is providing hands-on workshops for local people on how to start growing the no-dig way.

The action

In the workshop, participants learn how to construct raised beds and then how to mulch, plant and tend their crops. Bob teaches them the benefits of the no-dig approach, which include preserving energy otherwise used to dig, causing minimal disturbance to the delicate microorganisms and worms in the soil, and minimising the number of weed seeds that can germinate when dug up to the surface. Mulching is used instead to prevent weeds from growing, to protect the soil's water content and to increase the fertility of the soil.

The No-Dig Gardening Project is, however, much more than a series of one-off workshops. Instead, Bob uses the sessions as a way of creating a network of local gardeners, of encouraging the sharing of gluts, and of strengthening food security and production in the area. The wisdom of the following, slightly amended Chinese proverb has guided Bob in his work: 'Give a person some vegetables and you feed them for a day. Teach them how to grow vegetables, and they can feed themselves for a lifetime.' Bearing that in mind, part of Bob's mission is to ensure that food-growing skills are spread throughout the community, so he asks workshop participants to share their new-found knowledge with at least two other people they know.

Project name: The Master Chef Series

Location: Whitstable, Kent

Aim: To reskill local people with the foraging, preserving and cooking skills necessary to make the most of their local produce.

Started: November 2008

How many people involved: Three main organisers, one celebrity chef, approximately 100 audience members per event.

Transition initiative website: www.transitionwhitstable.org.uk

The idea

Once we have sourced our organic, local food, there is then a world of skills and tips that can teach us how to make the most of it – in terms of both taste and minimal wastage. Many of these skills have been lost and undervalued by our culture's reliance on the quick, 'convenient', processed food that has helped to banish creativity and cooking knowledge from our own kitchens. Abi Murray and the rest of the food group folk in Transition Town Whitstable in Kent have come up with an entertaining way of reigniting a passion for cooking and food preparation for local residents, framed within the context of food resilience. Two of the food group members were also the founders of the Whitstable Farmers' Market, so forces were joined to run a series of four Master Chef evenings, in winter, spring, summer and autumn respectively, each to be presented by an experienced chef and to focus on foods that were local and seasonal at that time.

The action

The first event was held in November of 2008, and featured TV wild chef Fergus Drennan, otherwise known as 'Fergus the Forager'. Fergus is known for promoting the virtues of free, wild food (see his article on page 40), as well as for inspiring much inventiveness in the kitchen. This 'feral food' will most likely play an important role in supplementing our diets in the energy-lean times that are to come, so now is a good time to start exploring what it is and how it can be used in our diets.

The event was sold out and attended by almost 100 community members of all ages. Throughout the evening they listened to Fergus's wild anecdotes and watched him create dishes using wild plants he had picked locally earlier in the day, including wild mushroom tabouleh, wild leaf-and-flower salads, hawthornberry squares and sea-buckthorn sorbet – all of which were tasted by audience members. During the interval, local breads and cheeses were provided by the farmers' market team, while local beers, ciders, juices and wines were available at the specially organised bar. A raffle was held for two spectacular food hampers – one containing delicacies specially made by Fergus; the other made up of a range of items donated by the farmers' market. The feedback received after the event was hugely enthusiastic, with participants commenting that the evening was "really inspiring" and "one of the best community events in years".

Initially, Abi and team paid for the costs of the venue hire, drinks for the bar, promotional and decorating materials, and for Fergus's time out of their own pockets. But they charged £8 for entrance fees to the event and also raised £120 from selling raffle tickets, so they managed to reimburse themselves while also making a profit of £220. This money was put towards the next event and used to subsidise ticket prices so that they remain low and accessible to all. Abi was particularly pleased with the raffle's success and puts it down to the fabulous prizes on offer – a high precedent that the team intends to match at their other events.

Following Fergus's wild evening, the second Master Chef event has been held with local chef Rob Cooper, who talked the audience through ways of using, cooking (and not wasting) all the different cuts from a local lamb. The Master Chef Series as a whole is a good example of how the necessity of reskilling be turned into an entertaining, tasty and fun community event.

Some words from skilled foodies

On the following pages are a few articles by food lovers and teachers that might help to inspire ideas for food reskilling workshops. Beyond what experts are able to offer, however, it is also a good idea to ask your fellow community members what food skills they themselves would be interested in learning, or indeed if they have any contacts who would be good workshop facilitators. These are questions that could be asked in an email, at a community event, on a feedback form after another reskilling workshop, or even on a blank sheet of paper posted up on a community noticeboard.

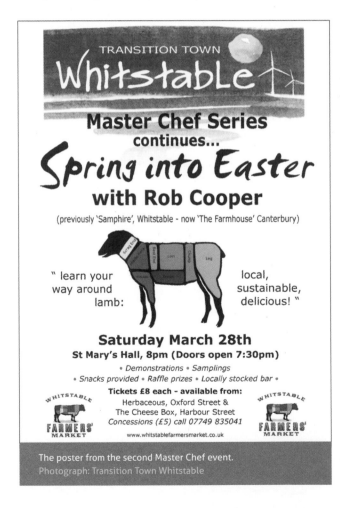

The poster from the second Master Chef event.
Photograph: Transition Town Whitstable

'Companion': the alchemy of bread making

Eva Bakkeslett

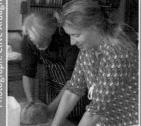
Photograph: Clive Ardagh

Food and land and labour and human dignity are the only real sources of value, but we trade those for cash hardly giving a thought for our children, our air, our water. But we can't eat cash, no matter how much we make! So the value of bread is not in the price, but in the inherent integrity of the cycle, from seed to grain to mill to dough, into my stomach and back out to the soil, via my composting toilet.

Kiko Denzer, *Build Your Own Earth Oven*

I was brought up in Arctic Norway where baking bread is still common in many homes. My grandmother and father baked bread, often in batches of six, so it would last a week. When I moved to England I brought my bread-baking traditions with me. The white substance you could buy in shops bore no resemblance to what I would define as bread, nor did it contain any of its qualities, so I simply had to bake my own. As my life and art amalgamated, my bread baking also became my art. I wanted to communicate bread making as poetry – as a way of reconnecting with nature and our senses. This became the film *Alchemy*, which has been shown in venues worldwide and resonated with its audience.

Baking your own bread is not only a wholesome and aesthetic experience but also a form of cultural activism. Here nature and human culture collude. By choosing your ingredients with care and being aware of the transformation of energy from the sun through the grains and sensing your own rhythmical movements in the kneading, bread baking can be a ritual that reconnects soil and soul. The timeless beauty of the process brings baking into the realms of poetry and becomes art that goes beyond the walls of the gallery and on to our kitchen tables. Everyone can become artists through sculpting, baking and sharing their bread.

The Latin roots for *companion* mean sharing of bread – *com* meaning *with* and *pani* meaning *bread*. In Russia they still celebrate companionship and hospitality by greeting visitors with bread and salt. Although Britain lost its popular bread traditions and skills a few generations ago, it is never too late to reclaim this ancient art. By baking our own bread we can activate our senses and share our cultural activism with others in the form of good and tasty bread that will nourish our bodies and souls. This is true companionship – with our fellow humans as well as our Earth.

Eva Bakkeslett is a Norwegian artist and 'bread activist' who has explored the interconnecting themes of climate change and food traditions in her work. See her Alchemy bread blog at http://poeticsofbread.blogspot.com, and see more about Sustain's Real Bread Campaign, which includes a directory of real-bread makers, course details and interesting articles, at www.sustainweb.org/realbread.

Eating wild food: the challenges, benefits and consequences

Fergus Drennan

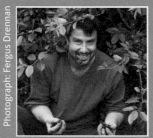

Photograph: Fergus Drennan

Eating wild food plants on a regular basis can improve your mental and physical health; diversify and enliven your daily menu; give you a really grounded sense of place; facilitate a deepening sensitivity to the environment; save lots of money; help you make new friends and, of course, facilitate spiritual enlightenment! Wild food defines who we are.

Throughout the vast sweep of human history, until relatively recently, our food has been none other than wild; our lives being orchestrated entirely by natural rhythms, the cycles and seasons, as we hunted, gathered and engaged in humanity's oldest occupation: foraging. Foraging wasn't the mere search for food but an all-embracing lifestyle based on a respectful and reciprocally positive engagement with nature. A healthy, vibrant and flourishing outer environment was contiguous with the health of one's inner world. Although we have mostly lost that connection (in part due to the unsustainable dictates of a fossil-fuelled existence), foraging is a way of relearning how to reap the benefits that flow from a direct and intimate communication with nature: a practical, experiential, environmentally responsive and exploratory conversation with the natural world and our proper place within it.

The great wild food adventure begins, of course, with plant and habitat identification, with the spring virility of the tree-sap harvest, the bliss of seaweed-searching seaside summer sun, autumnal mushroom mists and the frosty grubbing for winter roots. Of the A-to-Z of the hundreds of wild foods potentially available throughout the seasons many are simple to find, identify and prepare, while others require patience, persistence and a great deal of effort. Being skilled in the art of preservation and storage is also time-consuming, but deeply rewarding. Freezing, drying, pickling, bottling, brining, fermenting, smoking, etc. serve not only to preserve foods gathered at their seasonal best but also to provide the opportunity to create a colourful and kaleidoscopic range of foods unique in both texture and flavour.

For me personally, the greatest wild discoveries arise when going beyond simply substituting one or two ingredients in conventional recipes to eating nothing but wild food for entire days, weeks or months. The question then becomes how to get/make the essential and not-so-essential ingredients completely from scratch: bread, wine, salt, water, meat, flour, mayonnaise, houmous, pasta, vinegar, cakes – or, simultaneously, and more scientifically considered, how to obtain a healthy balance of protein, fat, carbohydrate, vitamins and minerals.

Take that biblically classic staple, bread, for example. In the absence of wild wheat, what and where are sustainable flour substitutes to be found – sweet chestnuts or horse chestnuts, acorns or rosehip seeds, reed-mace rhizomes or arum tubers? These are abundant resources, yet some are extremely toxic if not correctly processed when transforming them into flour, so research, experimentation and creativity are needed. No wild non-wheat flours contain gluten, so seaweed extracts can be incorporated into chestnut and acorn bread dough to provide sufficient structural integrity to hold the finished bread's crumb structure. Excess seaweed can be used for composting and the chestnut shells used for smoking seaweeds and other foods. Indeed, a sweet syrup can be obtained from the chestnuts prior to the solid residue being used to make flour, or acting as a chick pea substitute for wild-garlic houmous!

Foraging can be a joyful, reflective and deeply meditative experience either as a lone pursuit or in the company of friends. Indeed, working together helps to turn what may have seemed like wild food chores into seasonal acts of ritual and celebration, such as opening a tasty stash of dried seaweed or sipping a potent glass of sea-buckthorn juice collected months before. In company, foraging tasks can be completed in a fraction of the time, providing an opportunity for play and debate, as well as the experimental exploration of innovative and sustainable food projects. The small-scale, community-level extraction of high-protein leaf curd from the leaves of nettles, wild garlic, mallow and others is just one example of sustainable, wild food production that I am convinced has a crucial part to play now and in the future. A number of pioneers are already leading the way.

While foraging allows us to fully exercise our inherent creativity, imagination and sense of play, it does, like any activity, carry its own inherent risks. In order to feel vibrant and alive it is crucial, in the first place, that you remain alive. Following one simple rule will definitely help: don't consume any part of a plant unless you have identified the plant with 100 per cent accuracy; you know that the part you wish to eat is edible in the condition in which you've harvested, prepared or stored it; and you are sure that it is not contaminated with pollutants. With a wealth of traditional knowledge as well as a constantly growing database of scientific research to explore, such a rule has become both increasingly easy and, due to the sheer volume of research, difficult to follow. If, like me, uncertainty appeals to you as an integral part of the attraction of foraging, and you choose not to follow this rule as strictly as sense dictates, may I half-jokingly and half-seriously suggest that you publicly document your triumphs and catastrophes (assuming you are well enough to do so). That way, others may learn from your experience and potentially fatal mistakes.

Wild food use, to remain sustainable, must be seen as simply one aspect of the collective endeavour to live and eat sustainably. Through mindful foraging and other slow, low-impact and reflective ways of procuring our food (such as growing our own), we subvert the notion that food is a mere object or commodity, a barcode and bleep at the checkout, grown, graded, packaged, priced and distributed according to systems over which we have little influence or control. Foraging sustainably with an emphasis on quality over quantity, and food feet over food miles, can be seen as a radical act of rebellion against the current petrochemical-based systems of greed, excess transportation, packaging, waste and all-round general insanity associated with our industrial food system. By collecting just enough, just at the right time, just in the right place and with just the right company, foraging becomes an intentional act to embrace change and the eternal transition, with resilience, hope and growing wisdom.

Fergus Drennan is a chef, teacher and wild food forager, and the presenter of the TV series The Roadkill Chef *(see www.wildmanwildfood.com).*

Fermentation for food preservation, effective digestion and cultural adaptation
Sandor Ellix Katz

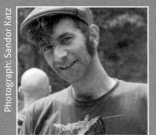

Photograph: Sandor Katz

One question that always arises when people in temperate regions think about shifting to a diet based on local foods is 'What do we eat during the long winter?' An important part of the answer to that question is fermentation, the transformative action of micro-organisms. Under proper conditions, bacteria that are present on all raw vegetables create acids that preserve the vegetables, improve their digestibility, augment their nutritive content, strengthen their flavours and protect them from contamination from pathogens. When we eat live (uncooked) fermented vegetables, we ingest beneficial bacteria by the billions, replenishing and diversifying important bacterial populations in our own digestive tracts.

Fermentation has always been part of human cultural evolution. The emergence of settled agricultural lifestyles makes no sense without fermentation techniques to preserve the harvest. Fermentation will be no less important as we revive local food systems and thereby liberate ourselves from dependence upon faraway food sources and fossil fuels for trans-portation and refrigeration.

Most of us consume fermented commodities on a daily basis. Beyond fermented vegetables such as sauerkraut and kimchi, there are beer and wine, bread and cheese, salami, coffee and chocolate, among many others. But most of that fermentation, like all aspects of food production, takes place behind factory doors. Because it is so hidden from view, and because of a growing cultural fear of bacteria, a great mystique has arisen around fermentation.

In reality, fermentation is simple and can be done in your kitchen without special equipment. Ancient rituals developed by our ancestors amount to simple manipulations of environmental conditions. For fermenting vegetables, it's a matter of submerging vegetables under liquid, usually their own juices, in order to protect them from exposure to air, which enables moulds to grow. Vegetables submerged under liquid always acidify and thus are intrinsically safe.

These are easy skills to learn, and fun activities for bringing people together and building community. Fermentation continues to provide us with the most effective means known to preserve food with nutrients intact. And the live-culture replenishment we get from ferments is more important than ever before, thanks to chlorination of water and overuse of antibiotics and antibacterial cleansers. Whatever changes the future will demand of us, fermentation will continue to be an important part of it, enabling us to preserve food with renewable resources, maintain effective digestion and good health, and embrace bacteria as our ancestors, allies and partners as we search for sustainable pathways toward a brighter future.

Sandor Ellix Katz is a fermentation revivalist and author, who travels widely teaching and sharing fermentation skills. His books are Wild Fermentation: The flavor, nutrition, and craft of live-culture foods *and* The Revolution Will Not Be Microwaved: Inside America's underground food movements. *For more information visit www.wildfermentation.com.*

Facing page photograph: istock photo

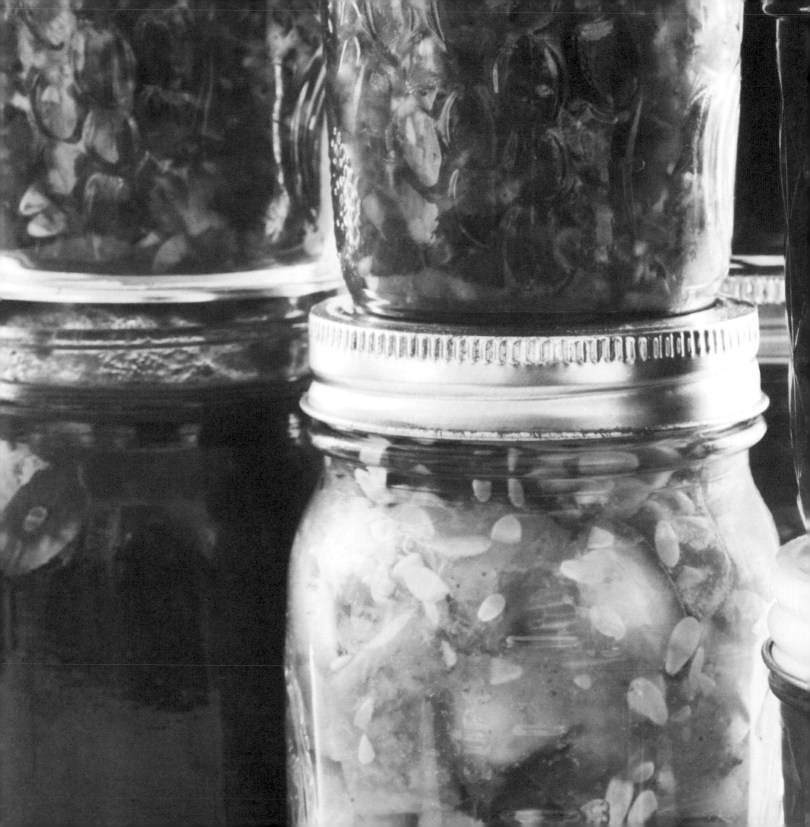

Preserving for a sweet future

Julia Ponsonby

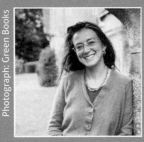

Photograph: Green Books

The preservation of seasonal fruits, alongside meat and vegetables, is one of the oldest culinary arts. Once practised as an essential skill for surviving during the cold, dark winter months when fresh food was scarce, fruit preserving has more recently become a specialist art employed for the treasury of lush flavours that jams, jellies, pickles and bottled fruit can bring to every meal, transporting it to the level of gourmet bliss.

Sun and wind were the first natural agents to be used for preserving food. Our ancestors discovered early on that fruits and vegetables laid out in the hot sun or hung in the wind to dry lasted longer than fresh produce. They were a great asset to a nomadic lifestyle, being lighter and more robust to carry than fresh food. In colder, damper climates, smoke and fire were used to speed up the drying process. Later a theory of preservation developed. Heat sterilisation destroys enzymes and bacteria, while drying or adding sugar, salt, vinegar or alcohol creates an environment in which contaminants are unable to thrive.

The use of sugar as a preservative is a relative newcomer to the business of conserving food. Cane sugar was introduced to Europe from the West Indies in the sixteenth century, and by the nineteenth century preserving had really come into its own as a skilled craft practised in most households. A generous pantry well stocked with bottles and jars of sweet preserves was a source of great pride. In the twentieth century preserving became less fashionable as imported produce, brought in on the wings of an oil-rich economy, made many fruits available all year round. By the 1960s and 1970s almost every household had a refrigerator and a freezer and this became the preferred, high-energy, low-effort way of preserving fruit and vegetables.

Today, as we transition back to a society that depends less on fossil fuels and less on imports, the challenge is to recapture our seasonal preserving skills. For optimum health benefits these must be married with our greater knowledge about the health risks that come with consuming too much sugar (such as obesity, hypoglycaemia, diabetes, high blood pressure, heart disease, tooth decay, etc.). The art is firstly to use sugar minimally and secondly to mix and match the techniques of dehydrating seasonal produce with bottling and jam making. Thirdly, energy-efficient fridges can be used to offset the lower sugar content in jams, using them as a store place after opening (with less than a 50 per cent sugar content, moulds will rapidly begin to grow once the preserve is opened and the vacuum seal broken). The conscious use of smaller jars, and not opening too many at once, will also help: in our household we easily eat a whole jar of grape-juice-sweetened jam in a week – long before it goes mouldy. We never need to refrigerate it.

Jam making without the addition of sugar is an old tradition dating back to a time when sugar was scarce, and such preserves have been rediscovered as health foods. Many such recipes from northern Europe, France and Germany are available in the book *Preserving Food without Freezing or Canning* (Green Books) – a compilation of recipes put together by the farmers of Terre Vivante in France. These jams employ fruit juices and bulk fruits such as pear and apple as sweeteners.

Dehydrators are going to be adopted more and more widely as we return in earnest to living with and loving the seasons – together with the onrush of the harvesting and preserving fever that comes with seasonal awareness. If we live in a sunny climate, then sun-dried apples and tomatoes will almost certainly give a more delicious flavour. But for those of us living in northern temperate climates, sun-dried is (at present) rarely an option, and the use of a simple dehydrator becomes a must to top up what can only otherwise be done on the radiator, in an airing cupboard, above a wood-burner or on the odd sunny day. Dehydrators often need to be in operation for 24 hours to dry food – but after that no further energy is required. So although in the short term they use far more energy than a fridge or freezer, in the long term they use significantly less. Dried food can later be rehydrated or eaten as a snack, such as apple rings or fruit 'leathers'.

A further method of preservation, which, at Schumacher College in Devon, we have become more and more adept at, is bottling fruit in the autumn months. We use Kilner jars with rubber bands – just as my grandmother did. Cooking the fruit sterilises the produce and then a vacuum seal is created once it is placed in the jar. Sugar (unrefined) is added only to taste. After opening, the apples and plums are usually eaten within a couple of days and kept refrigerated in between.

Moving from the home bottling of fruit to larger-scale canning, the drive to set up community gardens and community bakeries is now beginning to branch out into the setting up of community preserving kitchens.

These will become a social meeting-and-doing place of a very seasonal kind – where produce can be collectively or singly processed with the help of simple machinery that it makes sense to share. For someone with a small kitchen, keeping a large sauce-pan and fitting it on an average 60cm domestic hob can be problematic. But already organisations exist to share apple presses and other harvest-orientated equipment. The next step will be for shared processing spaces to evolve – and perhaps collective buying and storing of some of the less easily attainable ingredients such as salt, sugar, oil and vinegar.

Just as today we mix pleasure with good sense, and hope the latter will prevail most of the time, so in our localised future we will be doing the same. Some people will be encouraged to keep sugar entirely out of their store cupboards because of its increasing cost and the fact that it is an energy-intensive crop, while others will use it tactically for special preserves. When it comes to vitamin content, dried and bottled fruits are the winners – but, of course, jam is still nice when it comes to finding something to spread on your toast in the morning. Instead of telling children not to be too greedy with the chocolate spread, mums and dads will be saying 'Hey, hold off on the jam. Don't forget its made with *sugar*! A little goes a long way.'

Julia Ponsonby is the senior caterer at Schumacher College in Devon (the internationally recognised centre of holistic science and sustainability studies – see www.schumachercollege.org.uk) and the author of the award-winning cookbook Gaia's Kitchen.

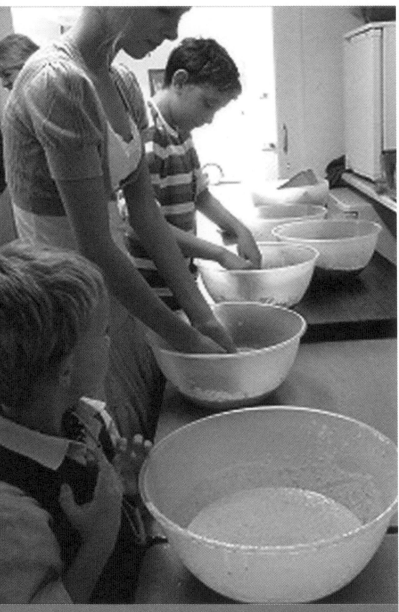

Community bread making in Glastonbury.
Photograph: Transition Town Glastonbury

Tips on holding Great Reskilling events

As suggested by Bob Jones (the No-Dig Garden Project) and Abi Murray (the Master Chef Series, Whitstable).

1. Make good use of the internet to advertise your reskilling events. Ideas include creating a special website, an event page on Facebook (www.facebook.com) or using Twitter (www.twitter.com) to post reminders about upcoming dates.

2. Make friends with local shops and businesses, and make sure they know that Transition initiatives support local economies and so it is worth their while to link in with Transition's work. You can benefit from these partnerships by advertising in their windows and promotional material, and by encouraging them to donate prizes to raffles and other fundraising efforts.

3. Use raffles to raise funds – they are a relatively straightforward but effective way of raising money at an event – as long as the prizes are wonderfully enticing, and, if possible, relevant to the theme of the event.

Resources

See page 201 for The Great Reskilling.

Chapter 3

HOME GARDEN GROWING IN THE COMMUNITY

The obvious place to start an investigation into local food production is home garden growing – quite simply, people growing food in their own gardens. While growing one's own food has been and still is fundamental to basic survival for many around the world, the availability of cheap energy and the growth of global trade over the last century has (in economically wealthy countries such as the UK) relegated edible gardening to the realm of disposable pastimes. But as the consequences of peak oil, climate change and economic recession converge, increasing one's own self-sufficiency is now being seen as less of a hobby and more of a necessity for greater numbers of people. We need only look to Cuba's recent organic food-growing revolution as an example of the important role gardeners can play in feeding a nation. The city of Havana produces more than 90 per cent of the fruit and vegetables consumed by its residents,[1] more than 100,000 of whom are gardeners trained to help run (amongst other growing spaces) 28,000 kitchen gardens or *huertos* across the city.[2]

The potential for home garden growing is significant. As Shaun Chamberlin points out in his book *The Transition Timeline*, the human-intensive labour involved in home-garden food production is hugely more energy-efficient than large-scale, mechanised agriculture, and to turn the UK into a nation of millions of food-producing gardeners would be a considerable boost to our food resilience, while alleviating the pressure on our local food networks.[3]

For those of us lucky enough to have an outdoor space where we live, growing fruit and vegetables at home is the cheapest and most energy-efficient way to put wholesome, fresh food on our families' plates. In permaculture terms, situating food-growing sites in the area or 'zone' close to the home and the centre of human activity is the most practical way of organising living space. Amongst other benefits, growing at home means that plants requiring high maintenance get the attention they need; there is virtually no cost in energy or fuel output in getting to and from the growing site; crops can be easily harvested as soon as they are ripe; kitchen, garden and water waste can be used to nourish the plants; and then there is the joy of being able to watch your plants change and grow day by day.*

The rise in allotment waiting lists (see Chapter 4) is of course indicative of a growing and wider interest in self-grown food – what could be seen as a silver lining to the cloud of difficult times. According the UK's Horticultural Trades Association, sales of seeds rose by 14 per cent between 2007 and 2008,[4] with food-producing seeds comprising up to three quarters of all sales for one seed retail business.[5] This is a trend that is echoed in other parts of the world. In the US, for instance, the National Gardening Association noted a 25 per cent rise between 2006 and 2007 in the amount Americans spent on growing their own vegetables.[6] Small-scale food production of the kind seen in

* See page 71 for estimates of how many people could be fed by cultivating all of the UK's home gardens for food production.

private gardens around the world will not address issues of food accessibility alone, but it is a crucial part of a larger effort to prepare for what Richard Heinberg calls 'peak everything'.

While home garden growing is an activity that doesn't always extend beyond the person or household tending the plants, there are a number of ways a community can work to link up the home garden growers in its area (and one would be hard-pushed to find a community in the UK, or indeed in many parts of the world, that didn't have any such growers). The following three projects are diverse examples of how these links can be forged, each one encouraging a sharing and proliferation of the knowledge, experience and practical examples of food growing that flourishes behind hedges, fences and walls.

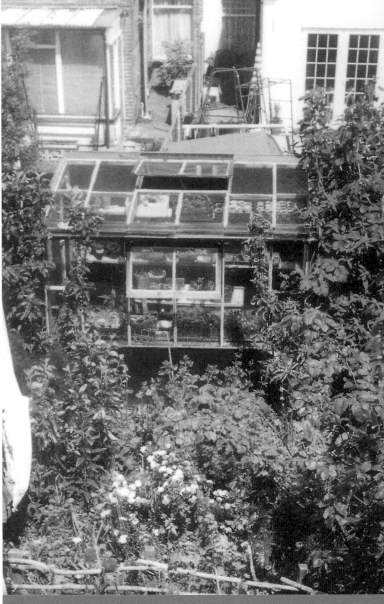

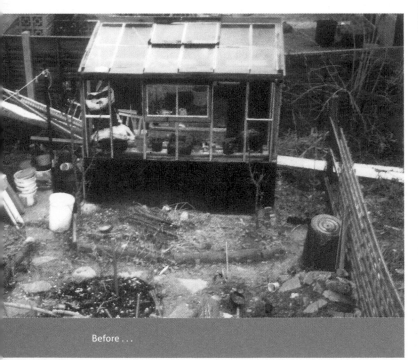

Before . . .

. . . and after Graham Burnett's garden had reached its full glory.
Photographs: Graham Burnett

Growing at home
Graham Burnett

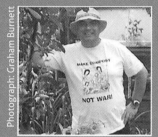

Photograph: Graham Burnett

We moved into our Victorian terraced house in Westcliff in 1994 and, armed with a copy of Graham Bell's *The Permaculture Garden* and leaflets from Plants For A Future (www.pfaf.org), set about developing the fairly typical north-facing 17x27-foot lawn, concrete path and drab flowerbed we had inherited. Our 'wants' from the garden included fruits, herbs and veggies to supplement our allotment, as well as a place that was aesthetically pleasing and attractive to wildlife.

Within eighteen months, the path had been broken up and used to make stepping stones and a rockery; we'd planted dwarf fruit tree and bushes; established vegetable, herb and flower beds; built a greenhouse from recycled wood and glass; dug a wildlife pond; made a worm bin and built a fence/climbing trellis to keep the children from the pond and more fragile crops. Early edible yields included lettuces, carrots, beans, brassicas, tomatoes, sweetcorn and quinoa(!). However, such annual crops became supplanted by perennials as the trees and bushes matured, e.g. fruit including apples, cherries, blackcurrants, quince and loganberries; and permanent 'sallets' such as lovage, sorrel, sea beet, Welsh onions, three-cornered leeks, Good King Henry, Turkish and wild rocket, lemon balm and so on.

The ethics and design principles of permaculture play an important part in our garden, but over the years I've also formulated these three 'golden rules' for the would-be food-growing landscaper or Transition horticulturist.

1. Don't overdo it. Keep within your physical and financial limitations. It's better to thoroughly develop a small area – probably not more than a few square feet for a beginner – than take on too much and simply exhaust yourself and your enthusiasm.

2. Take it easy. Observe, learn to fit in with the rhythms of the seasons, and take time to listen to the experience and advice of others. But don't let a lack of confidence or experience intimidate you into indefinite procrastination. You won't always get things right first time, but that's fine. Remember that the person who never made a mistake never learned anything either – and we've made our fair share.

3. Enjoy yourself! If creating a sustainable garden feels more like a chore than a pleasure, it's probably not worth doing in the first place!

I would stress that we are by no means self-sufficient from either garden or allotment, but neither is that our goal. Instead we prefer to think of ourselves as part of a self-*reliant* community by also supporting local shops, farmers' markets, box schemes, etc., contributing to local economic resilience just as much as reducing food miles.

Graham Burnett is a permaculture teacher and publisher, a member of Transition Town Westcliff and author of a number of publications including Permaculture: A beginners guide *and* Earth Writings *(see his website www.spiralseed.co.uk for more information).*

Home garden growing stories

Project name: Open Kitchen Gardens Project

Location: Lewes, East Sussex

Aim: A tour of local, edible gardens for town residents to promote home growing, make community connections and share skills, knowledge and ideas.

Started: Autumn 2008

How many people involved: Three main organisers, nine households, up to thirty-five attendees.

Transition initiative website: www.transitiontowns.org/Lewes

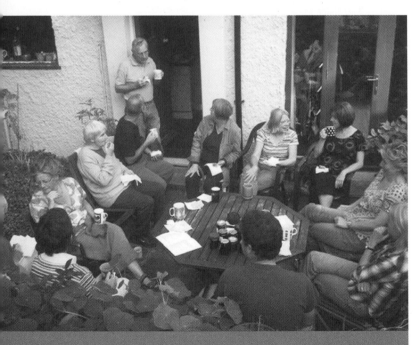

Participants enjoying tea in one of Transition Town Lewes's Open Kitchen Gardens. Photograph: Transition Town Lewes

The idea

Graham Burnett's description of his own back garden shows what productive abundance can be achieved over time, and in this case within the framework of permaculture wisdom and design. His is also an example of the rich inspiration that can lurk in private gardens – gardens that, if the owner is willing, can be used to help encourage other local people to convert lawns into vegetable patches and seeds into food.

Such was the thinking behind a recent scheme in Transition Town Lewes, East Sussex. Lewes is home to an active and progressive Transition group that, amongst other initiatives, launched its own local currency (the Lewes pound) in autumn 2008. The idea of the Open Kitchen Gardens project was to give other local residents the opportunity to see what fruit and vegetables their neighbours are growing and how they are growing them, and to spread awareness about why food growing is so important. It was also a chance for residents to meet and chat with fellow townsfolk sharing their interest in home-grown food.

The action

Transition Town Lewes's food group first explored the scheme in the early summer of 2008, when the group's coordinator, Polly Senter, opened her own garden gate to the public as part of a local open garden initiative. This gave the group an idea of how to plan for a larger pilot event, which they then held on a weekend day the following September. The event comprised a tour around nine private gardens and one public space, which was plotted on to a map and sold as a programme for £2.50. Polly and company worked to make sure they had a good selection of gardens making up a varied route around the town, and they advertised the event on the Transition Town Lewes listings and on posters.

The pilot went well. About thirty-five people attended and funds were raised from the sale of the programmes and teas, and donated through collection pots. A few days after the garden tour, the food group held a 'digestion session' where they mulled over what went well and what they could do better next time.

On the back of this pilot, the group intends to run the garden tour three times a year – in the spring, summer and autumn – so that participants are able to see, discuss and learn from the seasonal changes in the gardens. Garden tours are a relatively simple, community-strengthening way of accessing the immense knowledge, experience and deserved pride of home growers. They may also act as an inspirational springboard for others to start mulching their own lawns. But inspiration drawn from seeing others' edible successes is more likely to grow to action if people are given a helping hand – which is why a number of Transition initiatives and other community-based groups have begun running practical projects and courses on small-scale food production – see Chapters 2 (The Great Reskilling) and 5 (Garden shares) for more ideas. There are, however, also organisations that have emerged from, and are set up to serve and nurture, communities of home food growers. The following are two such organisations: they have developed replicable, fun and successful ways of encouraging the home-garden-growing approach to food.

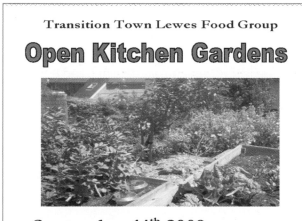

Transition Town Lewes Food Group

Open Kitchen Gardens

September 14th 2008 [2.00-4.00pm]
Entry by Programme
£2.50

Come and meet some new and some experienced gardeners and find out how to
'grow your own'
fruit and veg.

The programme from the Open Kitchen Gardens Project.
Photograph: Transition Town Lewes

Project name: Out Of Our Own Back Yard (Ooooby)

Location: Waiheke Island, New Zealand

Aim: To create a web-based network of back-garden growers, which can be used globally to promote local food events, food swaps, skills, knowledge, labour and ideas.

Started: 2008

How many people involved: Many, and more by the day!

On the web: www.ooooby.ning.com

The idea

Pete Russell has been working in the New Zealand centralised food industry for a number of years, but his growing awareness of the fragility of the

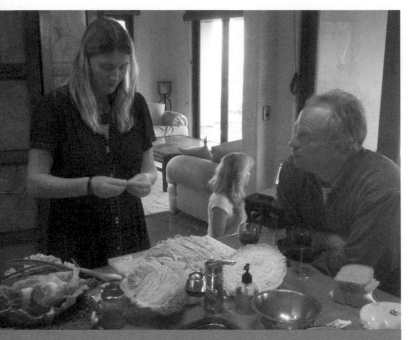

An Ooooby community dinner at Pete Russell's home on Waiheke Island. Photograph: Pete Russell

globalised food system and his family's dependence on it spurred him to start thinking about ways of mitigating a potential food-supply crisis. As Pete became more involved with his local Transition group on Waiheke Island he was inspired by the creativity and dedication that the Transition process was giving rise to, and began investigating organisational models that prioritised community well-being over the generation of profit. These new concerns compelled Pete to set up a social enterprise himself, with a name that brightens the otherwise dull world of business acronyms – Ooooby. Standing for Out Of Our Own Back Yard, the initiative is, according to its website, designed to "inspire, encourage and enable people to grow food and connect with other food growers", and it does so on many levels.

The action

At the heart of the Ooooby model is a web-based portal (see www.ooooby.ning.com) that is essentially a Facebook for foodies. Though it initially served the food-growing community of Waiheke, it is designed to be of use to a global network of home garden growers, and word about Ooooby has spread across the sea to Australia and as far as the UK. Anyone who signs in can create their own group specific to their local community, and encourage other residents to join them. Oooobites can then use the site as a way of sharing events, tips, tools, ideas, plans, videos and back-yard gluts. Because it is a web-hub, people who sign up can benefit from the wealth of information-sharing that happens amongst other food-growers across the globe.

In Waiheke Island, Ooooby has grown to incorporate regular events (such as Ooooby cuppas, where locals regularly meet to share their garden produce) and a recently opened Ooooby store (a venue for meeting, eating, swapping and learning). The group is also developing an alternative currency, known as Oollars. As the enterprise grows, all surplus money generated from the store or events that are held will be ploughed back into Ooooby and its community-building objectives. Because of its ability to draw communities together around the subject of local food, Ooooby is an idea that neatly complements the Transition concept (as it was designed to do), and it is Pete's vision that Ooooby can be used as a tool and model by Transition initiatives and other community projects worldwide.

Project name: Food Up Front

Location: South London

Aim: To train, support and link up back-garden growers.

Started: 2007

How many people involved: A team of two project coordinators and twenty-three working-group members.

On the web: www.foodupfront.org

The idea

Back in the UK, there are several organisations that are springing up to facilitate community engagement around home garden growing. One such project is Food Up Front (FUF), a London-based initiative that started independently of the Transition movement but that has recently supported and assisted a number of Transition Towns in and around the south-east. Before meeting on a permaculture course, Seb Mayfield and Zoe Lujic had each conjured up their own ideas of how to go about demystifying the food-growing process for others, while proving it was possible to grow your own on the smallest inner-city windowsill. A few months later, Kate Swatridge joined the team, having also entertained ideas of how to get her neighbours growing food. Zoe had trained in horticulture, Kate was a self-taught gardener and Seb was a keen novice, and between them they set about advertising their plan of assisting other inexperienced growers by handing out leaflets at their local farmers' market in Balham. The idea was that they would go round to people's own homes, give them a demonstration on how to get started, and provide them with pots (sourced from Freecycle), compost (from a local garden centre) and seeds (that they bought in themselves).

The action

In the early days the project was funded entirely by Seb and Zoe, and they were offering their services, time and materials for free. The initial aim was to recruit ten households, but more than fifty signed up – an encouraging sign that their project was tapping into a felt need in their community. Zoe, Kate and Seb did find, however, that only about half of the fifty households actually went on to grow and nurture their seeds to productive plants, so they decided that to ensure more of a commitment from their customers and to fund the growth of the project they would start charging people who wanted to sign up to the scheme. Making that decision has allowed them to develop their vision and roll it out to a wider area of South London.

Having evolved since its early, more informal days, FUF now consists of an Urban Food Growing network linking home growers across South London, a team of street reps responsible for dispensing materials and giving growing demonstrations and advice to nearby members, and a programme of workshops, talks and social gatherings throughout the year. At the time of writing there are sixty street reps in Balham, Wandsworth, Southwark and elsewhere, each of whom is the first port of call for new members in their street or neighbourhood.

The FUF team holds induction days for would-be street reps, and provides ongoing support to them in their roles. The aim is to make sure new members are within walking distance of their street rep, so that starter kits can be picked up on foot and explained face to face, and so that food-growing communities and social connections can be more easily established. As a result they have seen a number of food-growing hubs springing up around FUF's work – many of the participants share holiday watering duties, gluts, seeds, tips and all-important drinks evenings. The FUF team has also been amazed at the cross-section of people signing up to the initiative – from young city workers to retired older couples; from the unwaged to the well-off – and part of the beauty of the whole exercise has been in seeing relationships form across boundaries of age, race and class, and in a city where many people don't even know their next-door neighbours' names.

Zoe left the project in the summer of 2008, but Kate and Seb now run it between them. As the project evolves, they are becoming clearer about the structure of their organisation and how they want it to work. They have, for example, refined their role description for street reps and, on realising that being able to effectively communicate with new members is just as crucial as a practical understanding of growing, they have begun to emphasise social awareness in their rep induction days. The funding they received last year has helped to cover the costs of running FUF (though not the salaries – they are still working voluntarily), helping it to grow. Though they are currently dependent on this funding, their aim is to be financially viable so that they have enough members and can run enough fundraising events to cover the core costs and wages that their work requires.

As part of a recent effort to involve street reps in running and shaping the organisation, Kate and Seb have set up seven working groups, each focusing on a certain aspect of FUF's work, including those overseeing events, media and marketing, and finance. This has been an important move that helps to spread responsibility and decision-making more widely, gives the street reps a sense of ownership over the voluntary work they do and makes the project more sustainable by reducing the need for external funding. Part of their long-term plan is to find out how many

households could receive FUF support per paid full-time street rep coordinator – a model that, if successful, they hope to roll out elsewhere in the UK.

Beyond Food Up Front

FUF's success has attracted the attention of Transition Towns in South London because it provides a fun and easy way of encouraging home food production in the community. Establishing links between FUF and Transition groups is also a mutually beneficial way of strengthening grassroots action and community interaction in the area. An example of how the two initiatives can work well together was seen in Brixton, where the local Transition group decided to buy twenty memberships from Food Up Front to pass on to some residents at subsidised rates (this was done as part of a bigger community food-growing project on a local estate, detailed on pages 87-8). Kate and Seb have also done talks, workshops and joint events for other Transition Towns, including those in Tooting and further afield in Lewes.

Some closing thoughts on home garden growing in the community

Besides those projects listed in this chapter there are many other people working in communities around the world, encouraging their neighbours to get planting. There is, for instance, a movement currently sweeping the gardens of Melbourne, Australia, called Permablitzing (see www.permablitz.net for more information), where a group of local people get together with a trained permaculture designer and, in a blitz, create spaces for edible growing in private gardens (with the owners' full blessing of course!). No doubt more initiatives will continue to emerge from the desire and need to link up existing home growers and to make it easier for others to follow in their wellied footprints. In areas where there isn't already a thriving home-garden network or support organisation, these are simply opportunities and spaces that new ideas and actions can fill.

Tips on engaging community members in home garden growing

As suggested by Polly Senter (Open Kitchen Gardens Project), Pete Russell (Ooooby) and Kate Swatridge (Food Up Front).

1. Have a look at Graham Burnett's tips on page 49.

2. When it comes to gardening skills, read the books, do the courses, chat to fellow gardeners and don't be afraid to experiment! See page 200 for a selection of resources on gardening.

3. Stimulate conversations in your community around home growing, if only by transforming your front lawn into a vegetable patch, organising home-grown meals for friends or sharing your gluts with neighbours.

4. Create events where home growers can meet, network, share and have fun.

5. Be proud of your home-grown produce and show it off to friends, family and neighbours or as part of a garden tour. Awareness of the importance of home growing will spread most easily through social networking and community involvement.

6. If creating an organisation around home growing, spread responsibility and ownership between members as early on as is possible, and ask the fledgling gardeners you work with what they need from your organisation and how they'd like you to help them.

7. Encourage soil-based action by establishing a gardening book, tool, seed and compost share amongst neighbours.

Resources

See page 202 for Home garden growing, page 200 for General edible gardening, page 209 (More sources of help and interest) for permaculture resources, and page 197 for Funding, grants and loans.

Chapter 4

ALLOTMENT PROVISION AND GARDENING FOR COMMUNITY GROUPS

Allotment gardens exist in many parts of the world, from the UK and Germany, where they have a long, established tradition, to countries such as South Africa and the Philippines, where the model has recently been introduced. While their size, purpose and usage varies, they are generally described as being sites made up of small parcels of land (between 200 and 400 square metres to each plot) that are owned by local government or private organisations and rented separately to individuals, families or groups. According to the National Society of Allotment and Leisure Gardeners (NSALG) there are at the time of writing approximately 300,000 allotments in use in the UK, covering 12,150 hectares of land and with the capability of producing approximately 250,000 tonnes of fresh food each year.[1] They have an average annual rent of £29, though discounts are often available for those who are entitled to concessions. Plots are commonly 10 poles in size (a pole being an old form of measurement taken from the end of the plough to the nose of a local ox), which is equivalent to 250 square metres. According to the UK Allotments Act of 1922, allotment plots must "be wholly or mainly cultivated for the production of vegetable or fruit crops for consumption by the occupier or his family" – a legally ambiguous phrase which has led to varied interpretations in different allotment sites around the country, with some allotment holders being allowed to 'distribute' (including sell) their 'surplus' produce while others are not.

There are three types of allotment in the UK:

- Statutory allotments are council-owned, legally protected and can be taken out of use only with the approval of the Secretary of State.

- Temporary allotments are again council-owned but, lacking the same legal protection, they are vulnerable to selling for other purposes (such as the building of car parks, supermarkets, schools, etc.). Most allotments are either statutory or temporary sites.

- Privately owned allotments, held by individuals or organisations such as churches. Again, these are not protected by law as permanent sites for food cultivation.

While allotments were traditionally run by individuals and families, recent years have seen a growth in the number of groups expanding the definition of allotment 'occupier' and pooling resources, time and labour to cultivate shared plots. This is possible even when the tenancy agreement requires the signature and legal liability of one named plot holder. There is, therefore, some overlap between the categories of allotment described in this chapter and the community garden projects discussed in Chapter 6 – a small group of community members can, for example, take on an allotment plot between them and call it a 'community allotment', (in fact they can call it whatever they like!), or larger organisations can cultivate a number of allotment plots between members and volunteers (as done by the Organic Lea workers' cooperative in East London). Generally, however, the main intention with all these ways of running allotment plots remains to grow food for the consumption of the defined group, even when remaining gluts are shared, swapped or sold more widely. For the purpose of this book, those projects featured in the community gardens chapter (while they may perhaps be comprised of a few adjacent, council-owned allotment plots) can be seen, by contrast, as being bigger in scale and set up for use as a community resource on top of the aim to cultivate food.

In the UK, allotments have their roots in the history of access to land and food production – struggles largely triggered by the impoverishing effects of land privatisation for the landless many. The resultant reclamation or donation of land from private ownership to common access can be traced from as far back as the Saxon era, through to the tenanted allotments of Elizabethan times, and on to the General Enclosure Acts of the nineteenth century. These Acts attempted to ameliorate public resistance to privatisation, by establishing and protecting 'field gardens' for common cultivation – precursors to the allotments we now know.

In 1908 the Smallholdings and Allotments Act placed a duty on local authorities to provide allotments where a need is perceived for them in their area: a stipulation that has been upheld by subsequent Acts and is still in force today. As described in the introduction to this book, the threat to national food security at the time of WWII required a massive mobilisation of skilled and unskilled agricultural labour, and resulted in a huge uptake in the number of gardened allotments, peaking at 1.4 million plots in the 1940s.[2] Although existing allotment sites played an important role in the national efforts to relocalise food production, they couldn't provide enough of the growing space that was needed, and much creativity was required to try to feed communities across the country. Additional sites were established along the banks of railway lines, in public parks and in graveyards, and small-scale food cultivation was visible, vibrant and valued by the many that depended on it.

Apart from a brief resurgence of self-sufficient activity in the late 1970s, the uptake of allotments has steadily declined since the war years, as our reliance upon imported food and supermarket 'convenience' has grown. Sadly, this lack of interest in food growing, together with the pressures of economic growth, have meant a loss of allotment sites as they have been sold to make way for new developments.

But things are beginning to look brighter once more. In recent years, the revived interest in the ecological and personal benefits of 'mile-free food' has been reflected in the allotment waiting lists currently bulging in council offices up and down the country. While this renewed enthusiasm has seen previously derelict sites being restored to their former bountiful glories, it has also meant that, despite the optimism of the 1908 Act, access to allotment growing has been difficult for many. A University of Derby study in 2003 found that of local authorities surveyed, one-third of people on allotment waiting lists could expect to wait more than a year before securing a plot.[3] An article in *The Guardian* in March 2008 also reported waiting lists of up to 1,400 in Sheffield, 1,200 in Edinburgh and 1,000 in Plymouth.[4] There is clearly a gap between legislation and practice on the ground. But, as we shall see, some community groups have already had success in nudging their local authorities to provide the growing space their residents want and need. At the same time, more uncultivated, privately owned sites are being opened up for edible growing. The National Trust[5] announced in early 2009 that it is to make 1,000 new allotments available on its land,[6] which will provide much relief and joy for some lucky, list-weary gardeners. For those who are still feeling the weight of the many allotment-eager names above them, it is important to remember that allotment growing is one of many routes to accessing land and fresh, local produce – as the following chapters show, there are other routes out there.

Community groups can engage with allotment growing in a number of ways, from working to secure a plot to cultivating, eating and learning from it. Not only is group work of this kind a way of strengthening community bonds, but its focus – of establishing, preserving and nurturing allotments – is also of important community value. Allotment sites are, after all, hubs of social interaction and networking, where local residents are linked by a common interest in growing their own food. Those who partake in the growing enjoy all the health, social and nutritional benefits that allotment working can give. Research has confirmed what many allotmenteers already know – that working in community allotment projects and other growing groups leads to lasting dietary changes, a higher intake of fruit and vegetables among participants,[7] greater community integration and a deeper appreciation of the natural environment.[8]

The projects illustrated below vary in their aims, size and age, and together they give a picture of some of the ways allotment-based community projects can play a role in supporting local food networks.

Allotment stories

Project name: The Awaiting Allotment Society

Location: West Kirby, the Wirral

Aim: To represent the views of local residents on allotment waiting lists and to press the council to make more land available for allotment growing.

Started: September 2007

How many people involved: Three original founders representing more than 500 listed allotment hopefuls.

On the web: www.transitiontownwestkirby.org.uk/ accesstoallotments.htm

The idea

In September 2007, the small town of West Kirby on the Wirral peninsula was feeling the early rumblings of Transition. At one of the initial meetings, local residents Margaret Campbell and Daniel Wright found that they had a shared interest in allotments – or rather, the lack of them – in their area. They exchanged stories about their mutual frustration at local waiting-list times and their council's failure to comply with statutory regulations in meeting the rising demand for allotment plots. But instead of being deterred by the brick wall that faced them, they decided to scale it. There were at the time 400 people on the waiting list – a number that continued to grow, reaching 510 by November 2008.

The action

Initially, Margaret and Daniel decided to start a petition to press the council for more allotments in West Kirby, clearly stating in the accompanying letter that "We don't want to drive to an anonymous supermarket for week-old vegetables transported from intensive agriculture abroad. We would like to walk to a community area where we can share the experience of working to produce cheap, fresh and healthy food."

This petition was followed by two more from other local groups, and pressure on the council began to mount. In April 2008, Margaret and two other residents decided to set up the Awaiting Allotment Society (AAS) (affiliated to the Wirral Federation of Allotment Societies), with the aim of representing the views of residents on the waiting list. They drew in support already received from their petition work, and gained more recruits from Transition events held in the town. Their campaign has so far included a sustained effort to engage with local councillors over allotment provision, the attendance of relevant council meetings, a flurry of letters, the informing of local media, much detailed research, and the setting up of a resource webpage – all of which has been done voluntarily and without the help of funding.

The rewards

While the local council's Cabinet Member for the Environment came on side very quickly, AAS members have found other council officers more reluctant to deal with them. But, as Margaret observes, "We make their job more difficult, but we persevere anyway!" The group's resilient determination has seen progress in the shape of a council-led Allotment Strategy that allocated £40,000 to tackling the issue and to funding the new post of Allotments Development Officer. At the time of writing, council officers are preparing a bid for a three-year programme of funding for allotment provision, to the tune of £300,000.

The AAS continues to follow council proceedings closely, objecting to development strategies that fail to acknowledge the need for more allotment space, and generally making its concerns known and heard. It logs progress on its webpage, from the work it does on the West Kirby ground to the parliamentary responses to a national demand for more growing space. Also on the webpage are comprehensive lists of publications, links, and campaign documents that can be downloaded and used by other groups. The society's willingness to share its experience, research and resources means that this is an important project not only for the folk of West Kirby but also for anyone in the country setting out to tackle the national affliction of the 'allotment wait'. AAS is rightfully proud of its work. In fact, its main tip for others wanting to embark on a similar campaign is to look at its webpage on the TT West Kirby website – advice that would-be allotment growers would do well to heed.

Project name: The Transition City Allotment

Location: Canterbury

Aim: To build up a community around food growing, to learn growing skills, to engage with the practical dimension of the Transition process and to reconnect with the growing process and the Earth.

Started: January 2008

How many people involved: Five core members; up to six other part-timers.

On the web: www.transitioncityallotment.blogspot.com. See also www.transitioncitycanterbury.blogspot.com

Although the queue for allotments can be found in communities all over the country, this is thankfully not the case in each and every village, town and city.

One city where a budding new group of growers has managed to secure and cultivate allotments with relative speed and ease is Canterbury.

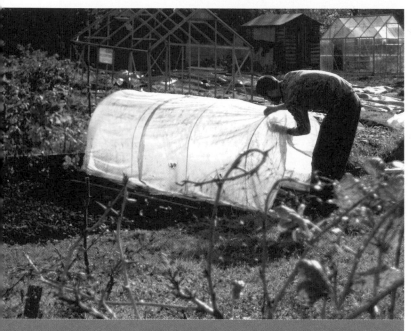

A spot of cloche care down on Canterbury's Transition City Allotment.
Photograph: Transition City Allotment

The idea

Towards the beginning of 2008 Transition City Canterbury began holding its initial meetings, where ideas were shaped, aired and shared. Local resident Kathryn Siveyer found herself in a food-focused discussion group and suggested the idea of starting up a community allotment. Kathryn had for some time liked the idea of taking on an allotment but had felt rather daunted by embarking on such a project alone. To do so in the company of other enthusiasts made the idea feel more possible. By the following weekend those

keen to be involved had (on the Transition City Canterbury grapevine), found out about an allotment site with free plots, checked out said (rather overgrown) plots, and decided to take them on. Because of the hard work that these plots required before planting and growing could begin, it was agreed with the site manager that the group would be allowed to use them rent-free for the first eight months.

The group was fortunate to have its allotment connections, via Transition City Canterbury, as this meant it could go directly to the site manager of the identified allotments rather than liaising with the local council over what was available and where – a process that would have been more lengthy. It was of course also lucky that the site location was suitable. George, the site manager (aged eighty, who has had a plot on that same site for no less than fifty years), receives the £24 of annual rental fees directly and sees to the management and maintenance of the site. It is the group, rather than the individuals within it, that is under contract for the plot, so responsibility is shared between all members. The plots themselves are also shared by the group as a whole, rather than being divided up and assigned to individuals.

The action

Now growing under the banner of the Transition City Allotment, the group is comprised of five core members, plus up to six others who pitch in when they can. Each member had some experience of home growing and they have a decent spread of gardening knowledge between them, but all had felt hampered by the limited size of their outdoor spaces. Being part of a community allotment was an ideal way of broadening their gardening horizons.

The first few weeks involved much digging, weeding, clearing and the inevitable bonding that comes with the sharing of hard work. Since then, the group has slipped into a more regular rhythm of group gardening. Sunday has become 'allotment day', and group members also try to meet in the week during busy growing times, to discuss plans and ideas for the next gardening session. They don't yet feel the need for a formal group structure or the assignment of roles – people simply gravitate to the jobs that suit them and they have enough space to accommodate the fruit and vegetable tastes of all group members. This relaxed, rule-less approach has so far suited the group well.

All necessary costs (including the site rental mentioned above) have been covered and shared by group members, so they have not needed to source any external funding. But expenses have been minimal, partly because they have received generous donations from the wider local community (including a greenhouse, tools, seeds and a wheelbarrow), but also because they are keen to be creative with what they have and what they can easily source. They have in fact been amazed and inspired by what they've been able to make and build out of very little, from tables to 'serious fortresses' protecting their broccoli. Fortressed broccoli aside, they are also growing blackberries, tomatoes, Brussels sprouts, leeks, raspberries, herbs, fruit trees and much more – the produce of which is shared between all members, with yields sufficient for Kathryn to make her own batch of jam from the first fruit harvest.

The challenges

The project has been, and continues to be, a productive, creative success, but there have been difficulties along the way. Of disappointment to some of the core group was the feeling that they would have liked more support and encouragement from other Transition City Canterbury participants – something they found frustrating in the first few weeks when the work was tough. It happens that in some Transition initiatives there is more of an interest in food growing than in others – but, as the Transition City Allotment team have shown, it is more than possible to build a successful community food project in a context where the same passions are not widely shared. Now the allotment has made such impressive progress, the group hopes that it will be acknowledged as a valuable, real example of a resilient approach to food production. It is now encouraging visitors to the plot, and inspiring them into growing their own food by sending them home with some seedlings from the plot's greenhouse. The group is also looking to recruit new members and entice more visitors through Transition City Canterbury seed swap events (see Kathryn's beautifully illustrated poster overleaf).

Down on the allotment the group has had to tackle other issues, such as organic pest control, the 'breathtaking rebuild' of a collapsed greenhouse and the realisation that two plots were more than the group could comfortably handle (one of these has since been passed on to a fellow Transitioner).

The rewards

While being able to eat allotment-grown food is of course a central part of the project, Kathryn is clear to point out that it is by no means the group's main reason for taking on an allotment. Of equal importance to the group is the growing of a small community, its reconnection with the Earth, and the building and sharing of new and old skills. The *way* these people are choosing to grow food (communally, organically, and with a willingness to learn) is, to them, as crucial as the mere act of growing it. Kathryn and others wanted theirs to be a practical demonstration of the Transition ethic – to show what delicious pride there is in moving from idea to action.

The group has many future plans for its plot, including developing a forest garden area and enticing frogs into the newly dug pond. As work develops, it documents its progress in words and stunning photographs on its blog (see www.transitioncityallotment.blogspot.com) for the bigger world

to see. The group's shared enjoyment of the experience is so evident that it seems likely their hope to inspire others to take up tools and do the same, in Canterbury and beyond, will be fulfilled.

> **Project name:** The Former LETS Allotment
>
> **Location:** Stroud, Gloucestershire
>
> **Aim:** To grow together as a group, providing fresh, mile-free, organic food for the group members' families.
>
> **Started:** 1996
>
> **How many people involved:** Seven households

We move now from a more recent, Transition-inspired allotment project to one that has similar values at its core but that was originally established in the nineties. The town of Stroud in Gloucestershire has been at the forefront of the local and organic food movement for many years and a number of its food projects have been a source of inspiration for others across the country. It could be said that groups in Stroud have been 'transitioning' by other names for some time, so Transition Town Stroud quickly took root in what was already fertile ground. The work of the Transition Town Stroud food group has therefore been as much about making links with some of the existing initiatives (including the following project) as about starting new ones.

The idea

It is in this setting that a community allotment has grown and flourished. Initially set up as part of the Local Exchange Trading Systems (LETS)[9] initiative in the area, the intention of the project was to grow fruit

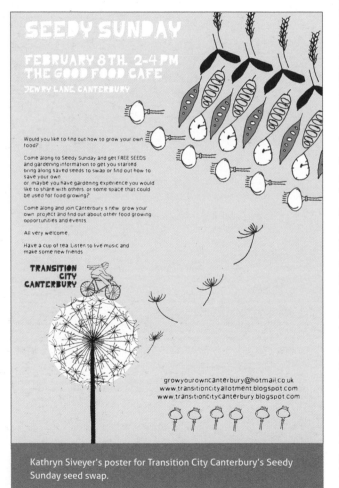

Kathryn Siveyer's poster for Transition City Canterbury's Seedy Sunday seed swap.

and vegetables for the families who would work on the plots, and to sell the surplus through the LETS scheme. In 1999 Sheila Macbeth joined the group that regularly worked on the allotment, and she has been a committed part of the project ever since. Though the LETS scheme in the area eventually crumbled, the core group of people that had come to regularly garden the plots each Friday morning felt committed enough to the project, and to each other, to keep it on.

The action

There are now seven households working on the four-and-a-half plots that are shared between this group of experienced gardeners. They grow organically, occasionally using biodynamic preparations, and the only digging they do is when turning green manure into the soil. Their situation is different from that in Canterbury, as not only are they required by their allotment committee to hold individual responsibility for each plot – so that five of the group are under contract for each of the four and the extra half plots – but they also have the pressure of waiting lists in their area. This means that should one member of their group pull out of the project, the others would have no control over whom the plot would be passed on to – it would simply go to the next person on the waiting list. So while the group has to accept that the project may not continue as it is forever, this does not deter its members from putting a great amount of care, energy and time into their shared garden for the time being.

The group in Stroud has been gardening communally for some time longer than the Canterbury growers described earlier, and in order to keep working efficiently and happily alongside each other they have found it necessary to settle upon a loose structure, routine and rhythm that works for them. But Sheila is quick to point out that the project is still 'gloriously free'

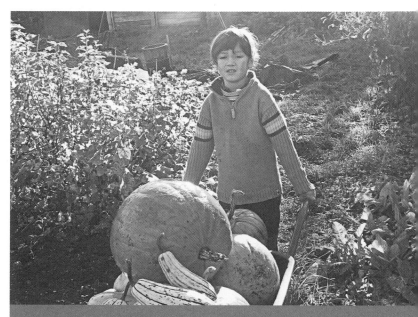

A younger member of the Stroud community allotmenteers showing off his gourd harvest. Photograph: The Former LETS Allotment

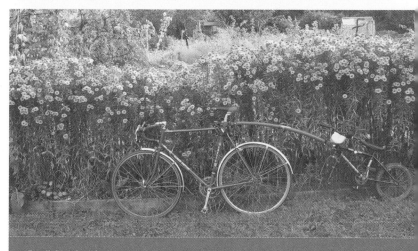

Fossil-fuel-free family transport to The Former LETS allotment in Stroud. Photograph: The Former LETS Allotment

of bureaucracy, box-ticking and committees, and that it is her hope it will remain that way. Post-LETS, the core group that kept up the running of the allotment eventually decided to make a commitment to keeping things at a size that suited all of their needs – which meant limiting the group to the seven households, the land to the four-and-a-half plots, and the scale of their tasks to one weekly work session.

The group pays its rental fees to the council who owns and administers the site. Of the seven households, four are waged and three are retired or low-waged, so they have decided to split the costs accordingly: the four waged households paying £33 a year into the allotment 'pot' and the other three paying half that amount each. Out of the total, approximately £30 is passed on to the council for its ground rent, and the rest is used to buy the seeds, potatoes, netting, tools and other equipment needed for the year. The group hasn't yet applied for any kind of external funding, and, for now at least, it is happy to enjoy the autonomy that this allows.

Friday mornings remain the regular gardening slot for group members, though times vary through the seasons – from up to four hours in the summer months to two in the winter. They try to manage the plots (with much mulching and little watering) so that they don't need to do any work between the Friday meetings, but during busier times (such as when harvesting the soft fruit) they may occasionally have to do weekend stints as well.

The challenges

Having first experienced shared, community gardening while working with VSO (Voluntary Service Overseas) in Papua New Guinea, Sheila has been struck by how much more individualistic we are in this country, and how much less accustomed to working in groups. To try to accommodate the group members' individual personalities, opinions and needs, they have, over the years, worked hard to strengthen the bonds within the group and to make space for the necessary discussions and debates that arise. They do this by scheduling a group coffee break during each working session, by meeting socially to have meals and to mark the pagan festivals, and by holding a traditional winter solstice lunch to review the year passed and plan the year ahead. They have also had to find ways to make communication between group members clear, such as having a blackboard to list jobs that need doing in order of priority, or using flags and signs to remind each other to help save seeds from the garden.

Sheila is clear to point out that community gardening is not without its difficulties – that it can at times make things slower rather than faster, that discussions can be lengthy and that personalities can clash. But the satisfaction that has come from remaining committed to the group, from working through the issues that confront it, and from trying to soften their own individualistic tendencies, means that they are all much happier working as they are than they would be growing alone. While their group gardening approach initially raised some eyebrows at the allotment site, they have more recently noticed an increase in the number of other gardeners sharing their plots and their workloads, particularly in pairs. The group's success has presumably been a source of infectious inspiration!

The rewards

Sheila is convinced that the group members are more productive as a community allotment group than they would be as individual gardeners. Her reasons for this are that different members bring a wider variety of skills to the group, there is more freedom for each

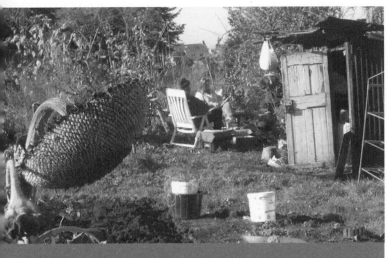
Nearing the end of an abundant summer on Stroud's Former LETS Allotment. Photograph: The Former LETS Allotment

become what is now an economically viable source of mile-free, fresh, nutritious food, demonstrating that community gardening is not only healthy and fun, but also financially sensible.

Project name: St Ann's Allotments

Location: Nottingham

Aim: To provide space for local residents and organisations to grow, enjoy and promote allotment-grown produce.

Started: The 1840s

How many people involved: Hundreds of people are regular growers, and many more visit or partake in projects on the site.

On the web: www.staa-allotments.org.uk

gardener to focus on the jobs he or she prefers, members have the security of knowing the plots will always be tended even if one of the families is away, and the company of fellow gardeners is a heartening source of encouragement for the work they all do. It also means that each family is able to take home a wide selection of produce, which might be harder to cultivate were they growing on their own.

Over the years, Sheila and the others have enjoyed a noticeable increase in the productivity of their garden, as the organic methods they use have improved the fertility of the soil. They are now in the happy position of having to work less for greater rewards. The group estimates that each household produces approximately half of its total fruit and vegetable needs for the year from the community allotment. Everything is shared between them, and they have managed to tweak their growing patterns enough to ensure they don't end up with huge gluts. The project has grown in efficiency to

Our last allotment story comes from the city of Nottingham, and focuses on a whole allotment site as a community resource and as a vehicle for encouraging local food awareness in the area.

The idea

St Ann's Allotments is the largest and oldest allotment garden in the world, having been established in the 1840s for city residents to enjoy and grow their own food. Since then it has seen and been a part of many historical changes, from a time when the majority of urban families had no choice but to grow their own food, through the 'Dig for Victory' campaigns of WWII, and to the more recent preference for supermarket rows over those of the vegetable patch.

The 75-acre site is made up of nearly 700 individual plots, still divided by the original hedgerows that the Victorians laid down over 160 years ago. Within the site is a community orchard, a number of community

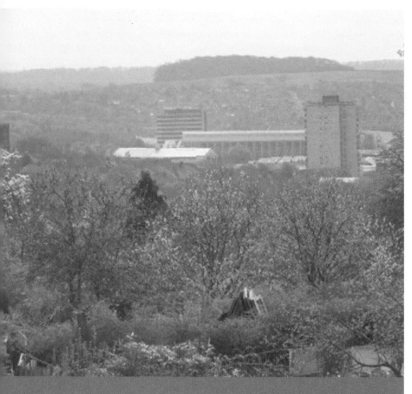

The view over the St Ann's Allotments in Nottingham.
Photograph: STAA

St Ann's and the threat of selling the site loomed. Now, in 2009, previously overgrown plots are nurturing food for local residents, there is a two-year waiting list, the site has become a Lottery-funded restoration project and it has received a Grade II English heritage listing, (affording it some protection from potential development plans). While a number of St Ann's gardeners represent a core of dedicated, experienced growers who have worked their plots for years, others have returned to the site having been re-inspired to grow food, and more people still are taking on allotments and entering the world of food growing for the first time.

The action

There are a number of ways St Ann's is and will be used to draw residents into building a more resilient community and city. Firstly, it is an ideal venue for learning: for holding workshops and training on food production and environmental awareness in general. Richard Arkwright is the coordinator of the St Ann's community orchard as well as a member of the Transition City Nottingham steering group, and has worked in the field of environmental education for years. He regularly holds workshops for children of all ages in the community orchard, giving them what is often their first contact with living, growing food. In a setting that buzzes with an enthusiasm for edible gardening, the children learn how to nurture seedlings, pick and press apples, build clay ovens and cook on fires – essentially, they receive what Richard calls 'a Transition education'. There are also a number of other events and workshops that happen on the site run by local organisations, including gardening courses, regular open days and community orchard activity sessions – all with the aim of opening up the gardens to the local community.

gardens, many plots cultivated by individual gardeners of mixed ages and cultures, and no less than three species of woodpecker! Management of St Ann's is now overseen by the non-profit-making company STAA Ltd, (St Ann's Allotments), who, among other tasks, work to make links with the wider community, conserve the natural environment on the site and promote allotment gardening in general.

In line with the national trend, Nottingham has seen a lengthening of allotment waiting lists in recent years. But, in only 2001, there were 200 vacant plots at

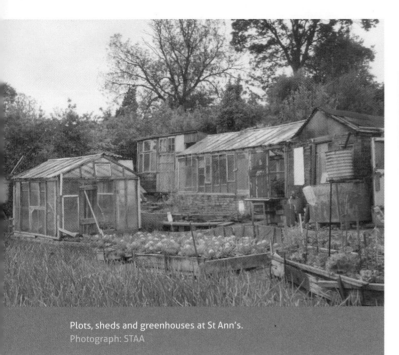

Plots, sheds and greenhouses at St Ann's.
Photograph: STAA

participants, and to thereby position food production at the centre of the city's Transition agenda.

> *It's not just about involving people in food growing, it's also about reconnecting people to their immediate local environment – as a first step to taking positive action to look after it.*
>
> Richard Arkwright, St Ann's Allotments

Secondly, St Ann's is a demonstration site that can be used to inspire others within the immediate community, Transition City Nottingham and beyond to start growing. The site acts as an entry point into the culture of growing food in the company of others, where people can see, smell, taste and feel that growing their own is both possible and beneficial. And amongst these 'others' there is a wealth of massed gardening experience that the less-experienced allotmenteers and the wider community can learn from.

STAA actively promotes St Ann's at community events around the city – for example, by running a popular stall and apple press at the Urban Harvest Festival in Nottingham in October 2008 (see pages 151-3). It is Richard's hope to be able to raise the profile of St Ann's among the network of Transition City Nottingham

Lastly, because of its rich history as a hub of food production, St Ann's is a crucial resource as a means of learning from the past. In acknowledgement of this, an oral heritage project was set up in the 1990s to collect and then to share stories from and about the site. The stories formed part of a roving exhibition that helped draw attention to the importance of St Ann's and its place in the city's unbroken history of locally grown food. The 'food feet' system that existed in this country prior to an increase in globalised trade was far more resilient and secure than the world-stretched supply chains that feed us today. St Ann's was a part of this kinder system and, because the site still survives, it can – through the work of the heritage project and through general publicity – be used to inspire a closing of the circle and a rejuvenation of the thriving, small-scale and local production of food that it was once at the heart of.

For all the above reasons and more, Nottingham is very fortunate to have St Ann's gardens preserved on the city's doorstep as a sanctuary for wildlife and gardeners alike. As such, the site is a good example of a wheel that doesn't need reinventing – that is, an existing, flourishing, hub of local food activity that the resident Transition group and novice food growers can tap into, learn from, promote and replicate.

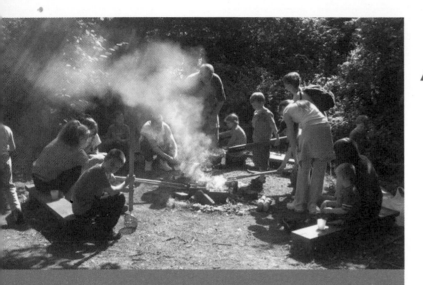

Popping corn on an open fire with local children at the St Ann's Allotment Community Orchard. Photograph: STAA

Tips on securing and running a community allotment

As suggested by Margaret Campbell (Transition Town West Kirby), Kathryn Siveyer (Transition City Canterbury), Sheila Macbeth (The Former LETS Allotment, Stroud), and Richard Arkwright (St Ann's Allotments).

1. If working to secure an allotment, check out the West Kirby website! www.transitiontownwestkirby.org.uk/accesstoallotments.htm

2. Be attentive to the small print on allotment tenancy agreements. Some will restrict activities such as coppicing, keeping livestock, having permanent crops or ponds.

3. If an individual is contracted as the plot holder that person will be legally liable for the whole group's activities, so there must be a sufficient level of trust within the group, and a clear awareness of what is and isn't allowed on the site.

4. Be sensitive to other allotment holders. Many can be apprehensive that gardening groups will disturb the peace or threaten the privacy of the site. Bearing this in mind, don't walk on other plots without the holder's permission, check with the allotment officer before having site keys cut for new members, accompany new visitors on to the site so others are not concerned they might be intruders, keep other plot holders informed of your group's plans and intentions, and if existing gardeners at the site are initially unwelcoming, be patient – they could well be a source of valuable support and knowledge in the future.

5. Security can be an issue on some sites, so be sure to either store your tools elsewhere or invest in a lockable container.

6. Watch 'Gardeners' World' and listen to Radio 4's 'Gardeners' Question Time'.

7. Forage in charity shops for second-hand gardening books to share between the group.

8. Be attentive to what others are doing on their plots and learn from what you see.

9. Try new things – there is much to be learned from exploring uncharted territory, as well as from the inevitable occasional mistakes that creativity brings.

10. Plan ahead and design your gardening space, as a group. Incorporate a meeting place or tea-break corner into your design.

11. Start small, and let your confidence and the project grow together.

12. From the outset, use mulch to cover as much of the plot as possible to protect the moisture of the soil and to keep weeds at bay.

13. Selling produce from allotment sites is a legal grey area and, on top of that, rules on selling also vary between sites. A very useful document that helps to explain the situation is available from Organic Lea's website – www.organiclea.org.uk.

14. Nurture the relationships within the group by holding regular social events, and by building discussion times into the group's routine. This will help to ensure the group can remain flexible and responsive to whatever may occur, to keep the channels of communication open, and to provide space for issues to be shared.

15. Be clear from the outset what the intentions are for the group – whether it will remain open or closed; whether decisions are to be made by a leader, democratically or by consensus; how jobs and produce are to be shared and assigned; and what gardening principles will be adhered to. Alternatively, agree that you are all happy for the group to remain formless and rule-free for the foreseeable future!

16. Use the many case studies and useful factsheets on allotment and community gardening found at www.farmgarden.org.uk/ari.

17. The National Society of Allotment and Leisure Gardeners provides much helpful information and support on how to secure an allotment. See www.nsalg.org.uk.

Tips on the role of allotment sites in strengthening community resilience

1. Make use of the knowledge and networks already established on the site. Other local residents will also be more likely to listen to and learn from them than outsiders.

2. Use allotment site noticeboards, newsletters and meetings to promote other community groups, projects and events.

3. With permission from the allotment committee, use the site as a place to run reskilling courses and workshops, and garden open days to inspire others to start growing their own.

Resources

See page 200 for General edible gardening, page 190 for Allotments and page 197 for Funding, grants and loans.

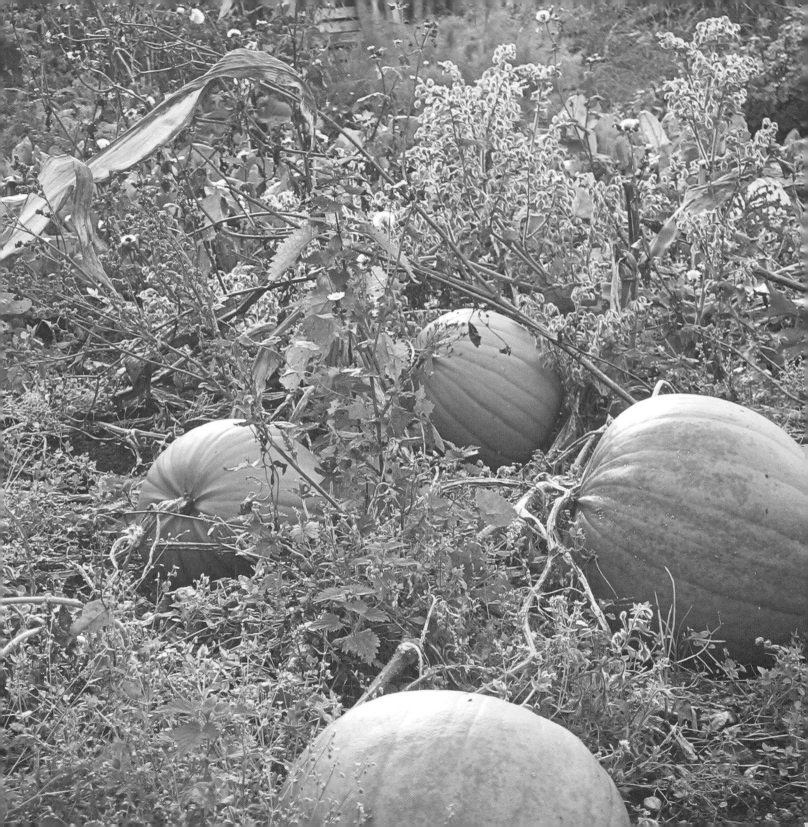

Chapter 5
GARDEN SHARES

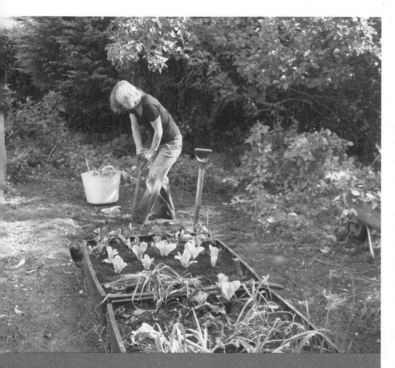

A garden share plot in the centre of Totnes, cultivated by Chris Watson and Trich Gilson and owned by a lady who was once one of Totnes' former master gardeners. Photograph: Transition Town Totnes

There are various estimates for how many private gardens we have in the UK, ranging from 10 million to over 20 million. Guesses as to how much land these gardens cover are just as wide – from 150,000 hectares to over 400,000 hectares (based on gardens having an average size of 190m²).[1] Taking the most conservative of these estimates (150,000ha), and figures suggesting that one hectare of agricultural land can feed between 7.5 and 10.6 people when farmed organically,[2] then the combined land area of the UK's gardens could potentially feed between 1,125,000 and 1,590,000 people. This is obviously a very crude calculation that doesn't take into account the quality of the land, the types of crop that produce the best yields, nor the complexities of the fact that one back garden growing a diversity of crops could potentially yield a greater total quantity of food than the same parcel of land within a large-scale, monoculturally farmed field.[3] But it does give a rough indication of the potential for home-garden food production that could be harnessed around the country.

When energy scarcity is a present reality, the mass-transformation of garden gravel, concrete, decking and lawn into productive patchworks of edible food plots will be a matter of necessity rather than choice. It will also require a great deal of community cooperation and a breaking down of private boundaries – a letting-go of our fondness for walls, fences and railings – if we are all to have access to the food we need. So one way of preparing for a leaner (and hopefully cleaner) future, while also creating a more healthy, abundant present, is to start to open up unused, private outdoor spaces to people

Facing page photograph: The Former LETS Allotment

who are keen and willing to start growing some food and who don't have access to their own land. By sharing our front and back gardens with others, we can do exactly that.

So-called garden share schemes work by match-making available private land (and its owners) with land-seeking others. They thereby help to put unused gardens to good use, while taking the miles out of food and forging links within the community at the same time. Garden owners partaking in these projects are keen to help local food-growing efforts in their neighbourhood and they either have spare plots alongside what they cultivate themselves, or, for whatever reason, they are unable to use their garden but are happy to let a neighbour tend the space instead. In return, these neighbours have a place to hone their gardening skills and grow their own food. With most garden share projects, arrangements are made between owners and gardeners that suit their mutual needs, so that some gardeners may pay a nominal rental fee, others may share part of their produce with the owners, and more still might have land access simply in exchange for the owner's pleasure in seeing food growing outside the kitchen window.

As practical solutions to land-access problems and the tedium of the allotment waiting list, it is not surprising that the popularity of garden share schemes has flourished in recent times, spawning initiatives such as the Tavistock Garden Share Alliance, the Isle of Wight's Adopt-a-Garden scheme, London's Capital Growth project (see Rosie Boycott's Foreword) and Hugh Fearnley-Whittingstall's Landshare website (see Hugh's article opposite). Transition initiatives have been enthused by the garden share concept too, and groups in Falmouth, Cambridge, Lewes and Farnham (among many others) are busy shaping similar schemes to suit and serve their local food-gardening needs – which means that there is already a wealth of garden-sharing experience across the Transition Network (in and beyond the UK) from which others can learn. Apart from simply making sense, these 'open allotment' projects represent a refreshing and radical shift towards prioritising community well-being over individual ownership, and trust over suspicion of our neighbours. In order to make sure this sense of trust is well protected and respected by all participants, many of these schemes have devised ways of safeguarding the rights and interests of all involved – an important aspect of the service that garden share projects (acting as 'mediators' between owners and gardeners) are able to provide.

As discussed in Chapter 2 (The Great Reskilling) and Chapter 6 (Community gardens), making more land available to food growers is only one part of a larger effort to avert a food crisis – it is also crucial that people have ways and means of developing the skills they need for edible gardening. By offering (or at least signposting) courses, workshops or buddy-gardener training alongside the garden share schemes, organisers make their project more accessible to a wider audience of would-be growers, while also helping to ensure that participant gardeners have the bountiful successes they aim for. Linking the scheme to a local food network, via a Transition food group or other relevant projects and organisations, can also provide more skilling-up opportunities, as well as facilitating access to other sources of support – such as outlets for surplus produce, food and seed swaps, tool shares and a community of local food supporters. Below are two approaches to sharing private gardens that have sprung from Transition initiatives and that are helping to reduce their communities' dependence on oil-fuelled food.

Sharing land, community and food

Hugh Fearnley-Whittingstall

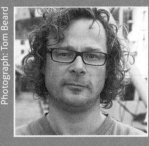

Photograph: Tom Beard

Growing a few potatoes in a back garden, tending a little fruit tree, perhaps digging a shared allotment patch – these things don't sound particularly revolutionary or innovative, do they? But these small acts of domestic agriculture can be part of something exciting, progressive and, if you'll excuse the pun, ground-breaking.

For decades now, we have been moving away from the land, away from self-sufficiency, away from even knowing where our food comes from, let alone growing it ourselves. That leaves us with significantly less power, less influence and less knowledge when it comes to choosing the food we want to eat. It leaves us heavily reliant on large-scale producers, often in other countries, and on massive commodity crops – which, if they fail, leave nothing in their place. And of course it means that much of the food we eat comes freighted with a rather large environmental price tag.

Sourcing your own food locally whenever you can is a simple way to redress the balance. Producing some of it yourself is even better, in my book. Combining these two approaches by working cooperatively with other local people to grow fruit and veg is perhaps most exciting of all – because you're not just feeding yourself. Such cooperative schemes help to sustain a whole community. And if the family that eats together stays together, just imagine what the community that eats together can do.

Garden share schemes are now cropping up (literally) all over the UK. The Landshare project is one I'm heavily involved in myself. We know that many people who want to grow their own food struggle to find the land they need to do it. Landshare brings together people with land to spare (anything from a postage-stamp back garden to a few acres) and people who want to start digging and planting. The scheme has already met with an incredibly enthusiastic response, and in back gardens, rooftops, car parks, derelict plots and country estates all over the UK people are taking small but incredibly important steps towards a more sustainable, secure, vibrant and varied way of producing food. Such projects are living proof that the future of our food is in our own hands.

Hugh Fearnley-Whittingstall is a writer, broadcaster, chef and campaigner committed to promoting seasonal, ethical food. He is the author of The River Cottage Cookbook *and many other publications, and presenter of the* River Cottage *TV series (see www.rivercottage. net and www.landshare.net for details of his own garden-share-inspired scheme).*

Garden share stories

Project name: Transition Town Totnes Garden Share Project

Location: Totnes, Devon

Aim: To link growers with unused land, establish community connections and build local food resilience.

Started: December 2007

How many people involved: One to two organisers, twenty-one gardeners, ten garden owners.

On the web: www.totnes.transitionnetwork.org/gardenshare/home

The idea

When Lou Brown joined the Transition Town Totnes (TTT) office team in 2007, she was encouraged to create and run a Transition project of her own, and, as a keen food-producing gardener and supporter of local produce, her thoughts immediately turned to the world of food. In the past, Lou had seen a garden share scheme turn disappointingly sour because of a lack of clarity between owners and growers, and this gave her the idea of setting up a project that could instead facilitate thorough, open and trust-based communication between the two parties. That way, misunderstandings wouldn't distract from the more important tasks of increasing land access and decreasing food miles for local growers.

The action

For the first couple of months, Lou had the voluntary assistance of a local lady called Lin Scrannage, a valued cohort on the project, and together they bounced ideas around, devised ways of protecting the rights of owners and gardeners, and drew up the necessary documents (discussed below). It was agreed that Lou's TTT wages would cover the time she spent on the project, which has so far been run without any other kind of external funding. One of the first steps was to advertise for garden owners so TTT would have something to offer the gardeners when they came to the scheme. Up went Totnes Garden Share Project posters, and out went TTT newsletter blurbs and a press release calling for people who had available garden space to offer to a local grower. Offers began to come in and Lou's matchmaking lists were opened. Once she had a good selection of plots, she then advertised for gardeners to take them on.

The way it works

On the phone or in person, owners are asked to fill out forms detailing the land they have to offer (including its size, aspect and condition, and available water, compost or storage facilities) and their expectations of the scheme (including what times and days they'd be happy for the gardener to have access, whether they'd mind more than one person working the plot, and what proportion of the harvest they'd like to receive in return). They are also asked to provide photos of the site to share with potential gardeners. At this point Lou outlines the scheme in full to the owners, to make sure they understand the commitment they are making.

Lou then goes through the same assessment process with gardeners who get in touch, asking them to come for a meeting in the TTT office to chat through their expectations, hopes and needs for a garden space, as well as their levels of gardening experience – all of which is recorded on a gardeners' form. This part of the process has become self-selecting, in that some potential gardeners drop off the list because they realise they don't actually have the time or enthusiasm to see the project through. Only those who are wholeheartedly committed to the scheme and to working within its necessary boundaries end up pursuing their land-seeking hopes to the final hurdle.

Those that do stick with the process go on the matchmaking list, and it is then Lou's job to pair up well-suited owners and growers, bearing in mind what times and days work for both, what gardens are within walking distance of a gardener's home and what expectations and hopes coincide. When she thinks she has a found a good match, Lou gets in touch with the gardener and owner in turn, and, without revealing any personal details, describes their potential garden share partner. She also shares photos of the garden with the would-be grower. If both sides are happy to go ahead, Lou gives them each other's contact details and leaves them to get in touch. As long as each is happy with the match, gardener and owner sign the garden share certificate (a written agreement to respect the other's rights and needs, downloadable from the website). Part of this agreement states that gardeners are committed to sharing a portion of their harvest with the owners, which is usually set at a quarter of the week's produce. They are also asked to sign up to the roving insurance policy held by the local organisation South Devon Community Supported Farming (CSF) which, for £7-10 a year, covers them for public liability insurance and can help to put owners' minds at rest. Lastly, the owner receives a garden share sign that, if he or she is willing, can be put up outside the garden so that passers-by will find out more about the project.

Lou calls up the gardener a week later to check how things are progressing, and gets back in touch every so often to make sure all is running smoothly. At the end of the season gardeners and owners are sent feedback forms to keep a check on participant satisfaction, and at the end of the scheme's first year all were sent back with glowing responses, confirming it to be a resounding success.

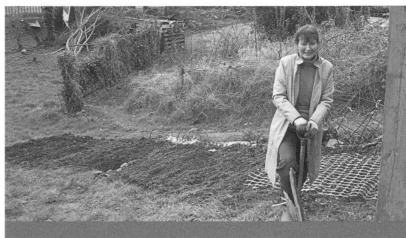

Sue Holmes on her garden share plot in the early days of its use.
Photograph: Transition Town Totnes

The rewards

One particularly content garden share grower is Sue Holmes, who joined the scheme because she no longer had access to her own garden and was eager to get her hands dirty once more. In her first year of garden sharing Sue estimates spending no more than £30 for the annual insurance, the cost of the seeds (which were available to buy cheaply at the TTT seed swap) and two large cloches. And yet for this small cost she has managed to transform a bramble-covered patch of land into a productive edible garden, satisfy all of her own vegetable needs between May and November, and to also provide two or three bags of vegetables and bunches of cut flowers to the garden owners each week. With the garden share sign pinned up outside

Sue's adopted plot the idea has spread, and there are now two further gardens in the same street (as well as others around the town) that are also part of the scheme and this growing Totnes community. Sue's garden hasn't just inspired other growers in her home town but those across the nation too, since it was featured on Hugh Fearnley-Whittingstall's TV series in 2008. Hugh and his team were in fact so impressed by the scheme that they set up their own nationwide Landshare project, which works on the same principles of matching gardens and gardeners but on a larger scale and via the web (see Hugh's article on page 73 and www.landshare.net for more information).

gardening courses. Participants attribute much of the success to Lou's thoughtful planning and infectious enthusiasm, and to the fact that she has made gardeners and owners feel that they are respected and valued members of the garden share community. Many participants are thrilled to be keeping physically fit, making new friends, sharing skills and contributing to a stronger sense of community in the town. Lou is herself very pleased that the scheme has provided fresh, seasonal, local food for up to fifty people (gardeners and owners combined) within a relatively short space of time, and that everyone involved has been so dedicated, creative and conscientious in their respective roles. While she points out that the garden share is just a small part of a bigger local food picture, its popularity, steady growth and national ripples of success have extended its relevance far beyond the gardens it has helped to nurture. All the necessary documents and suggested guidelines for setting up a similar project are available for download from the TTT website (see www.totnes.transitionnetwork.org/gardenshare/home).

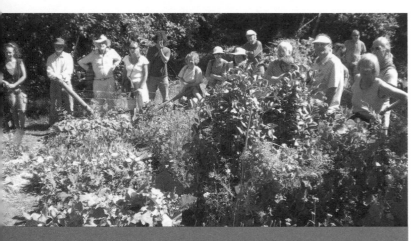

Sue Holmes's garden share plot later on in the year, being proudly shown to onlooking participants of the edible garden crawl.
Photograph: Transition Town Totnes

At the time of writing the Totnes scheme has more than twenty-one active growers and ten gardens participating. It has also held an edible garden crawl around some of the plots, and a number of basic

Project name: The Travelling Garden Group

Location: Kapiti, North Island, New Zealand

Aim: To support back-garden growers in the community by holding group work sessions in private gardens every fortnight.

Started: August 2008

How many people involved: Twelve regulars, forty less-frequent participants.

Transition initiative website: http://ttk.org.nz

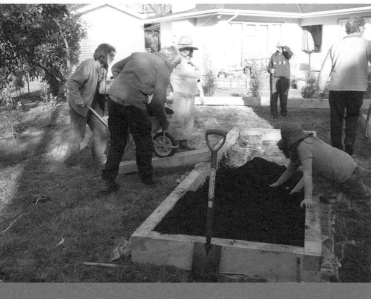

The travelling gardeners get to work in Kapiti.
Photograph: Transition Town Kapiti

The idea

This project, run by Transition Town Kapiti (on the south-west coast of North Island, New Zealand), is a variation on a garden share theme. It too provides an effective way of opening up private gardens to wider community access while pooling the skills and labour of local growers. The idea grew from an Open Space[4] event run by the Transition group in July 2008, which focused on how to strengthen food security in the area. In response to an observation that community gardens weren't taking off too well in Kapiti (as most people there have their own outdoor space), participants came up with a project that could work within the context of private gardens while still nurturing community spirit. The following month, Transition Town Kapiti's Travelling Gardening Group was born.

The action

The gardening group meets fortnightly at the home of a different group member. Its purpose is to help him or her work on the garden, to share knowledge and ideas, and to build a network of growers in the area. Andrew Rundle-Keswick, who helped establish the group, was thrilled to have ten people working in his garden for two hours at one of the first meetings – twenty person-hours in return for refreshments felt like a worthy exchange. Together they built a raised bed using blocks from a recently chopped-down phoenix palm, prepared an area for a forest garden, weeded, drank tea and coffee, and had a good gardening chat.

In 2009, the group is made up of a mixture of experienced and novice gardeners, with a core of about twelve who regularly participate and up to forty others who dip in when they can. Their mailing list enables them to advertise the details of upcoming sessions among members, and they have an online question-and-answer forum which means they can pursue a cyber-conversation between meetings. The project has required no funding, has been relatively simple to set up, and continues to be an effective way of providing support and encouragement to the new and established food-producing gardeners of Kapiti.

Some closing thoughts on garden shares

If you decide that some form of garden sharing is the thing for you and your community, you can either go about organising your own independent project, as Lou and Andrew have done, or link in with an existing regional or national project (such as the Tavistock Garden Alliance or Landshare respectively), depending on what suits your group and how much time and energy you have to commit to the idea. Either way, garden sharing can help to stimulate edible growth in your home village, town or city, and encourage others to trade in the supermarket trolley for wellies and trowels; the strip-lit aisles for the tranquillity of the garden.

Tips on setting up a garden share scheme

As suggested by Lou Brown (Transition Town Totnes Garden Share Project) and Andrew Rundle-Keswick (Kapiti's Travelling Garden Group).

1. Make all participant responsibilities clear from the outset and put safeguards in place (such as contracts, insurance, etc.). This way you can allay any possible worries about starting a project that requires such levels of trust. By emphasising that part of the project's aim is to break down the modern-day culture of fear, you can encourage people's willingness to cooperate to shine through.

2. Give participants regular opportunities to air grievances, or work through any garden share issues by calling up participants every few months, and by sending out feedback forms each year.

3. Encourage bonding between participants by holding regular social events such as picnics, garden-grown pot-luck dinners or garden parties.

4. Give non-participants in the wider community a chance to see what the project has achieved (and recruit more people in the process) by putting up eye-catching signs outside participating gardens, holding garden tours, putting articles in the local press or running a garden share glut stall at a local market.

5. Keep the project large enough to make a significant contribution to the community's local food network but small enough that it can be manageably run and participants get to know one another well. (Deciding what is too large or too small in a particular setting is something that only the organisers of a particular scheme can do.)

6. Access to ways of developing gardening skills, if not already incorporated into the scheme itself, is an important accompaniment to garden sharing. Organise one-off or ongoing gardening courses with local, experienced growers (see Chapter 2 for some ideas), link in with organisations already offering similar courses in the area (perhaps garden share participants could get a discount off course fees?) or list places that offer them locally on a handout for participants.

7. Have an email mailing list and online forum for participants – great for sharing tips, advice and news between participants.

Resources

See page 199 for Garden shares and page 197 for Funding, grants and loans.

Chapter 6
COMMUNITY GARDENS

Community gardens exist around the world in as many varied forms as the combination of people and land will allow. They can include anything from a shared greenhouse to a small-scale farm tending livestock; from a guerrilla-gardened floral roundabout to an education centre for socially excluded young people – but they all have the common factor of being run and maintained by members of the community. Many community gardens, though not all, focus their energies on food production as a way of bringing local people back to the earth and closing the gap between the plant and the plate. These gardens have a particularly important role in urban settings, where residents would otherwise have little access to green space or the process of food cultivation. They can also link in with existing local food networks, helping to supply market stalls and local shops, or act as a distribution point for co-ops or box schemes. In countries such as the US, where they do not have the same tradition of allotments as in the UK, some so-called community gardens are essentially what a British gardener would recognise as allotment sites – a patchwork of plots, each rented and cultivated by an individual, family or group.

Community gardens are established on whatever suitable land is available, whether leased from private owners or councils, squatted, or bought by the community group and turned into Land Trusts.[1] In the UK, the Federation for City Farms and Community Gardens lists 249 community gardens among its member projects, but there are estimated to be many more besides, so that the total number is likely to be more than 1,000.

While more and more community gardens are being established with the permission and cooperation of local authorities, some have been at the centre of contentious land struggles. This is particularly the case in cities where land is scarce and where the less-quantifiable value of community worth often finds itself up against the lure of real-estate profit. The original precursor to these modern-day land struggles was played out more than 350 years ago in the town of Weybridge, Surrey, when a group of hungry locals known as the Diggers began cultivating food together on land that had been privatised by wealthy landlords. Though they too were eventually forced from the land, theirs was one of the first attempts to reclaim the 'commons' from the landlords who had enclosed them, and it was a radical act that has been a source of inspiration for land struggles ever since – not least because of Gerard Winstanley's eloquent prose that defined and led the Diggers' movement:

Action is the Life of all and if thou dost not Act, thou dost Nothing. So I took my spade and went and broke the ground upon George Hill in Surrey, thereby declaring freedome to the Creation.

Gerard Winstanley, 1649,
A Watch-word to the City of London, and the Army[2]

Back in the present, some community gardeners today decide to bypass land ownership issues altogether by taking it upon themselves to 'illicitly cultivate someone else's land' – often in the dead of night and by torchlight. Known as 'guerrilla gardening', this method can, if done in a way that's sensitive to any existing plants and wildlife, help to turn neglected, unused land (and every community has some) into islands of edible abundance (see Richard Reynolds article opposite for more on guerrilla food production). One example of a community-based project that has embraced the guerrilla method is that run by the Incredible Edible Todmorden team from the Yorkshire town of Todmorden, where cherry trees have sprung up in supermarket car parks and leeks in the grounds of the local college (see www.incredible-edible-todmorden.co.uk for more information on its many other activities).

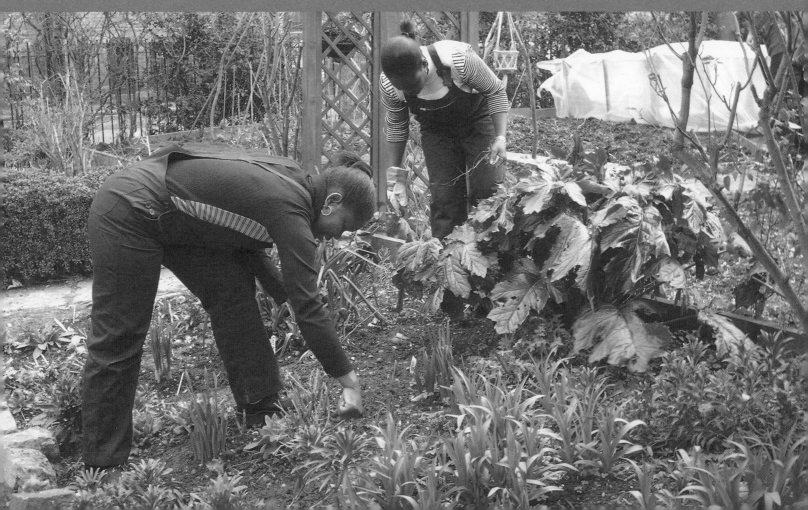

A thriving community garden in Hackney, London. Photograph: Hackney City Farm

Guerrilla gardening for food
Richard Reynolds

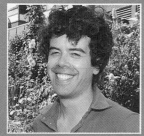

Richard Reynolds in front of his first guerrilla garden.
Photograph: Richard Reynolds

If you are a very enthusiastic vegetable grower, perhaps one without a garden with sufficient space or who wants to imaginatively alert the public to the productive potential in the land around them, then guerrilla gardening is for you.

Land used by guerrilla gardeners is usually public and, in the mind of the guerrilla at least, is not being put to good use. An abandoned flowerbed, a scruffy verge – places like this that are 'orphaned' are best suited to guerrilla activity because their negligent owners are less likely to notice or care. It can be an effective precursor to gaining permission, achieved through creative positive action and an assertive demonstration of personal commitment.

Guerrilla gardening is a growing movement across the world and includes both discrete individuals as well as more official groups that seek to sow a fertile proselytising message. The motivation to garden illicitly and risk prosecution for criminal damage, (which, incredibly, is the law on this matter) is wide-ranging: from simple local beautification to deliberate political provocation, in which plants become symbolic martyrs in what is usually a temporary vegetative display.

If you garden with equal measures of optimism and pragmatism, the law is unlikely to be a problem – though there is unfortunately a risk that your crop could be poisoned from pollutants. You can test the soil with a science kit but if the results are bad, all is not lost. Land can be cleaned naturally – sunflowers, for example, help remove lead from the soil and can be burnt or buried – and there is a powerful and positive symbolism in growing vegetables for their ornamental benefits. From the colourful foliage of Swiss chard, kohlrabi, rhubarb and red cabbages to towering canes of runner beans with their orange flowers and fruit trees with their spring blossom, our common land could be both tastier and more beautiful.

Richard Reynolds is a veteran guerrilla gardener and author of On Guerrilla Gardening: a handbook for gardening without boundaries *(see www.guerillagardening.org).*

Despite continuing and familiar tussles between community groups, landowners and developers around the world, a recent surge in awareness of the value of community gardens is helping to persuade increasing numbers of local authorities to preserve, create or support spaces in which communities can grow their own. This awareness has been given a high-profile boost by the American first lady Michelle Obama, who recently pledged her support for community gardens in a speech to the US Department of Agriculture employees.

> *I'm a big believer in community gardens, both because of their beauty and for their access to providing fresh fruits and vegetables to so many communities across this nation and the world.[3]*
> Michelle Obama

Michelle's own digging efforts in the famous, newly established White House organic vegetable garden will hopefully inspire thousands, if not millions of US citizens to start growing food, both in community and home gardens. Such was the case in 1943 when the then first lady Eleanor Roosevelt dug her own edible 'victory garden', sparking the establishment of nearly two million vegetable patches up and down the US.[4]

Supporters of community gardens cite the numerous benefits that these open, green spaces can have for a local area, not only for the health of those that engage with the project (in terms of nutrition education, physical exercise and social integration) but also for that of their immediate and wider environment. Indeed, a study carried out by the Federation of City Farms and Community Gardens found that 80 per cent of community farms and gardens surveyed had seen biodiversity increase on the site since their project was initiated.[5] Food-growing community gardens can help to reduce their community's dependence on fossil fuels by growing organic food on people's doorsteps and, crucially, they can provide city residents with the living, vibrant proof that food production can be an integral part of modern urban life. They are also perfect places for people to try their hands at gardening for the first time (as Patrick Whitefield points out in his article opposite, gardening skills are the most important output that community gardens can currently offer), where they can build up their skills before taking on an allotment or creating their own patch at home.

The community gardens described here are all dedicated to growing food, but they are otherwise varied in their shapes, aims, settings and more. As mentioned in Chapter 4, those featured in this chapter are larger in scale than the allotment growing groups described there, and have the added, outward-looking dimension of operating as a community resource – as a place that can be visited, tended, used and appreciated by the wider community. The colourful abundance of community gardens that exist around the globe is the context in which the following four projects sit, as they pull together Winstanley's vision ("Worke together, Eat bread together; declare this all abroad"[6]) with a modern understanding that we must learn to work and eat within the limits of this Earth.

Community gardens – filling the skills gap

Patrick Whitefield

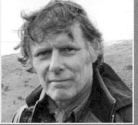

Photograph: Patrick Whitefield

The main output of community gardens is not food, at least not at this stage in the Transition process. It's gardening skill. Food is an important output, and lots of people who get involved in community gardens do so because they want to grow food but haven't got a garden of their own. But I reckon more people get involved because they want to grow their own but haven't got the skills. Faced with a back garden of wild, unruly grass or neat, bordered lawn, the prospect of turning it into a bountiful plot of delicious vegetables may seem a little daunting. Standing there with a gardening book in one hand and a trowel in the other, the inexperienced gardener may be pardoned the odd quake at the knees. Evening classes may add a human element to the cold impersonality of a book, but by far the best way to get started is by actually doing it alongside other people, fuelled by the conviviality and sense of shared purpose you get in a community garden.

If I close my eyes and imagine a resilient future I can see people everywhere tending their productive plots, bursting with abundant fruit and vegetables. There are many rivers to cross before we make that vision a reality, not least the shortage of land in many urban areas. But the deepest and widest of them all is the skills gap. It's the gap between the last generation, which knew about gardening as a matter of course, and the next one which will need to. The Transition movement is here to fill that gap.

Patrick Whitefield is a gardener, permaculture teacher and author of the books Permaculture in a Nutshell, How to Make a Forest Garden *and* The Earth Care Manual. *He lives, gardens and teaches in Somerset (see www.patrickwhitefield.co.uk).*

Community garden stories

Project name: Kinsale's Transition Community Garden

Location: Kinsale, Ireland

Aim: To create a community garden for local residents to learn how to sow, grow and harvest food, working together with others in a group.

Started: 2006

How many people involved: four to five facilitators, numerous volunteers.

On the web: www.transitiontownkinsale.org/projects/community-garden

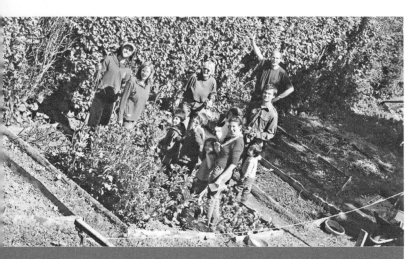

Kinsale's Transition Community Garden.
Photograph: Transition Town Kinsale

The idea

Dan Zev Benn's first introduction to community gardening was at the Whitehawk Community Food Project in Brighton (a more detailed description of which follows on page 88). There, volunteers work on the permaculture-inspired site in return for a share of the day's crop – an arrangement that to Dan felt like "the best thing in the world". Some time later in 2006, Dan was in Ireland studying on the Practical Sustainability course at the Further Education College in Kinsale, West Cork (the same course that Rob Hopkins set up and taught on). Transition Town Kinsale was just being unleashed, and Dan and others were keen to link up their permaculture skills with the emerging initiative. Through a series of fortuitous events and with the encouragement of the local Transition group, Dan and other students were able to secure funding for a roving community garden project. This was designed to be a modular course where participants from the local community could learn about all the elements needed to create a productive garden, held in a different back garden each week (an idea not dissimilar to Kapiti's Travelling Gardening Group, described on pages 76-7).

The action

As the roving garden course got under way, word of the project spread among local residents, and it was not long before a permanent piece of land was offered to Dan and company – a private back garden that wasn't wanted and that was slowly turning into a local refuse site. This became the permanent base for the project. The course continued to run (though it ceased to rove), and with the help of volunteers and course participants the rubbish tip was soon turned into a community garden complete with raised beds, a shed and a communal seating area. Once the funding had run out, Dan and others did their own fundraising at quiz nights and other events, in order to keep the community shed stocked with the necessary tools and materials. They based their project on the Whitehawk model, holding a weekly, open work session each Sunday where volunteers were able to come along and work in the garden in exchange for some of the bounty.

The Sunday sessions still continue today, though Dan has passed on coordination of the garden to others. In between Sunday meets, the site provides a space for courses and workshops on gardening skills such as mulching, fruit-tree growing and composting. Once a community group has such a space, the scope for using it is as boundless as creativity itself, and the Transitioners of Kinsale will no doubt continue to come up with new plans and ideas to win more local residents to the site, and to the value of local food production.

The challenges

One of the hardest aspects of running the project has been in making sure there is always an experienced gardener present when work is being carried out. This was of course easier when the funding covered the role of coordinator, but it is harder to maintain when all coordination work is done in voluntary time – especially at the busier times of the year. Because of the unpredictable nature of open sessions (these may pull in anything between one and fifteen volunteers), such a person or group of people is important for overseeing the work and ensuring that no overzealous weeding occurs. While the coordinators need to hold the project and keep to the design, they also try to accommodate the wishes and ideas of other users in the garden, by planting certain crops on request or taking cuttings so plants can be grown at home.

The rewards

Some volunteers may turn up regularly while others come only for a one-off experience. Those that do attend frequently have more input and ownership over the garden, and are of course rewarded with greater shares of the fresh, mile-free food they have helped to grow. As a way of cementing the social connections that are made during these sessions, some of the core volunteers have also started to follow their gardening work with a well-earned drink at the local pub.

Project name: The Glastonbury Community Garden

Location: Glastonbury, Somerset

Aim: To encourage healing and reskilling through the communal growing of food.

Started: October 2007

How many people involved: One main facilitator, numerous volunteers.

Transition initiative website: www.transitiontowns. org/glastonbury

The idea

One of the earliest towns to follow in the Transition footsteps of Kinsale and Totnes was Glastonbury in Somerset. Since 2007 the town has been active in promoting and building the concept of community resilience, and, perhaps because of its agricultural setting, there has been a particular flurry around the subject of food. As a practical person keen to see the Transition vision happening on the ground, Ingrid Crawford decided to dedicate her time to setting up a community garden in the area. Having lived in a community that grew its own food together, and having attended a permaculture course run by Patrick Whitefield, who lives nearby (and whose article on community gardens can be seen on page 83), she felt ready to put the word out on the Transition grapevine that she was looking for a site for the community

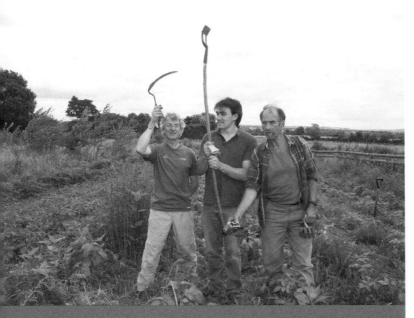
Volunteers at the Glastonbury Community Garden.
Photograph: Ingrid Crawford

project. At the same time Caroline Barry, a local resident very supportive of the aims of Transition, decided to make an acre of her land available and rent-free for community initiatives, so it was not long before the two of them got together to discuss plans for a community garden. Soon after, and having secured a start up grant of £250 from the organisation Somerset Community Food, the first work began on the site in October 2007.

The action

Community gardens have a long tradition of providing supportive learning and opportunity to people on the margins of society – one glowing example of this being Catherine Sneed's work with prison inmates in San Francisco.[7] Ingrid, too, is convinced of the healing that occurs when people engage with the alchemical process of growing food and when working in the company of others. Her project has therefore been driven by a firm belief in the transformative power of working with the Earth, and of the amazement and joy that comes in nurturing plant life from seed to food.

Determined to help those who could benefit from this experience gain access to land and growing skills, Ingrid linked up with local charity the Robert Barton Trust. She was hired by the Trust to train six of the individuals it supported – people experiencing social exclusion of some kind through circumstances such as job loss, homelessness or substance misuse. At the community garden they were given the opportunity to learn about food production, to cooperate as a working group, and to develop a sense of pride in their contribution to the project.

After the initial phase of clearing the site and preparing the beds with the Robert Barton volunteers, Ingrid opened the garden up to the wider community with weekly open sessions every Saturday, advertising through the Transition group and in posters put up around the town. The project attracted up to twelve volunteers at each session, and on the whole there were enough hands to cover the work that needed doing.

From the outset, (and together with financial help from the start-up grant and wages paid by the Robert Barton Trust), Ingrid has managed to run the project single-handedly and under her own steam. The erratic nature of the open-session approach means that it has been necessary for her to plan the garden and make overall project decisions herself, which has suited the volunteers well – many of them being complete beginners drawn to the opportunity of working with others but under the guidance of an experienced grower.

The rewards

Ingrid has been thrilled by the number of volunteers who, having encountered the magic of community-garden growing, have felt confident enough to begin cultivating food at home, or even to change their lifestyle to make time for food production. The Glastonbury Community Garden's successful first growing season culminated in a fabulous crop that included French purple beans, sprouts, kale, beetroots, carrots, spinach and chard. Anyone who came up to the garden to help was given the chance to pick what food they wanted, and there was always enough to go around.

Caroline has recently reclaimed the original site for other purposes, but Ingrid is in the process of securing a new plot and will continue to run the project. Her vision is to get more people on to the land, particularly those who are disadvantaged or who live with disabilities, and to see more local residents taking up the rare but growing opportunity to put time aside for working and gardening together.

Project name: The ABUNDANCE project (Activating Barren Urban Niches for Daring Agricultural Networks of Creativity and Endeavour)

Location: Brixton, London

Aim: To create a demonstration site of community, urban food growing on a Brixton housing estate.

Started: November 2007

How many people involved: One permaculture teacher, three main organisers, ten to fifteen volunteers.

Transition initiative website: www.transitiontown brixton.org

The idea

Not all community gardens are as fortunate in popularity as Ingrid's project in Glastonbury – sometimes, trying to convert local residents to the benefits of food growing can be like pushing a full wheelbarrow up a steep, muddy slope. But that is certainly no reason not to try! In November 2007, some Transition Town Brixton participants decided to raise the profile of agriculture in the area, having been inspired by the remarkable success story of urban food production in Havana, (as documented in the film *The Power of Community*). They soon found a site in a local housing estate (a former allotment area that was neglected and in danger of being landscaped), teamed up with University College London's Development Planning Unit, secured funding from the College's Urban Buzz scheme, and were ready to go. The Transition Town Brixton folk also got in touch with a permaculture teacher living on the estate, in the hope that the connection would open up doors within the estate's community. But, despite holding open meetings to pull residents into the project and to plan work for the community garden, few showed much support for the plans and their involvement was limited from the outset.

The challenges

According to Transition Town Brixton participant Duncan Law, the vision for the project was to achieve real partnership with estate residents and to work and plan in cooperation with them. But the TT Brixton team have found that, although they are local to the area, being 'outsiders' to the estate has presented them with a community hurdle – it is of course hard to instigate participatory planning if the community is not present to participate. Disappointed but undeterred, they have tried to drum up enthusiasm through leaflets, events and by working with the organisation Food Up Front (see Chapter 3, page 53).

In hindsight, Duncan and others recognise that the ABUNDANCE project would have benefited from a greater amount of community work before they took to their spades – more time spent knocking on doors, talking to locals and seeing what other organisations and groups they could have linked into. It would also have been a great help to have lived on the estate and been a part of the community there – or alternatively, to have found a suitable site in their own area. They suspect that if the community on the estate had felt ownership over the project from the beginning, designing and building it would have been a more integrated experience, and issues such as access to tools and roles of volunteers would have been clearer and mutually understood. In settings where the community is relatively closed (as is common in urban areas), it can take a great deal longer for new ideas to develop and be embraced, so it is hoped that over time the now-existing community garden will be valued and used by more of the people who live around it.

The rewards

While the original, community-engaged ideal is yet to be fulfilled, the project has taken the group down some unexpected but positive paths. As well as some dedicated residents who now regularly work on the site, a number of volunteers from surrounding areas have come forward, donating much time and effort to the garden. The project has in fact generated a great deal of outside interest both from the media and other initiatives wanting to roll out similar ideas, so the very act of *trying* to actualise the vision has inspired an increasing awareness of the aims and purposes of urban growing at large. And, although there were times when people-power was lacking, the garden produced a reasonable first crop of organic vegetables, and will hopefully continue to do so.

The community gardens described so far are projects that were initiated relatively recently, and that have emerged from community groups and a determination to start preparing the ground for fossil-fuel independence. As with the allotment-growing groups described in Chapter 4, these projects may well grow or take on more form as they develop over time and through the input of different community members. Brighton's Whitehawk Community Food Project, described below, is an example of one such established community garden with experienced, committed growers, strong community ties and a philosophy that binds the two.

Project name: Whitehawk Community Food Project

Location: Brighton

Aim: To allow local residents of all ages to engage in organic and biodynamic growing and to enjoy the garden and the production of food.

Started: The 1990s

How many people involved: Management committee of four members, numerous volunteers.

On the web: www.thefoodproject.org.uk

Started in the 1990s on a formerly disused area of an allotment site, this productive, edible sanctuary now covers over an acre on Whitehawk hill, overlooking the city and the sea (and situated right next to Transition relaxed and open to being shaped by the people that share the site. Although open sessions can be unpredictable, the experienced gardeners work to incorporate the views, ideas and suggestions that volunteers come up with, broadening the ownership of the site and the day's activities as much as possible. They often try to end the day by cooking and eating together on the site, and they also hold regular events and open days that include communal walks, talks, picking, cooking and even yoga classes. Over the years they have secured the odd grant, or done their own fundraising, but on the whole it is the management committee members who run the project in their own unpaid time, each contributing about two-and-a-half days a week.

Some closing thoughts on community gardens

Community gardens such as those described above can be a valuable, nourishing resource for local residents and wildlife. If sites like these continue to inspire more residents to start up their own allotment or community food projects (as did Dan Zev Benn and many others), then we can think of community gardens not as finite initiatives but as important spawning grounds for the kind of proactive, edible creativity that our food culture needs.

See overleaf for tips on setting up a community garden.

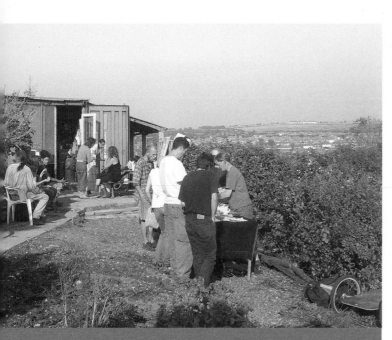

Feeding open day visitors at the Whitehawk project's community kitchen. Photograph: Tamzin Pinkerton

City Brighton's recently secured community allotment). The site is home to polytunnels, ponds, chickens, fruit, vegetable and herb beds, an orchard area, a community kitchen, and a large, covered, seated area for community feastings.

Two work sessions are held on the site each week, on Sundays and Thursdays, when members of the Brighton public have the opportunity to learn about organic and biodynamic growing alongside more experienced gardeners. The project has a firm commitment to community participation, a principle that the group members try to adhere to through every aspect of the site's maintenance. They have a management committee that is voted in at the AGM (open to all workers and volunteers) and meets up to four times a year, but on the whole their approach is informal,

Tips on setting up a community garden

As suggested by Dan Zev Benn (Transition Town Kinsale), Ingrid Crawford (Transition Town Glastonbury), Duncan Law (Transition Town Brixton) and Bethan Stagg (Community Scientist, Totnes).

1. Work hard to develop community ownership over the project and be creative in how you draw in other local residents. Some ideas for events to hold at the site include music festivals, treasure hunts, pot-luck meals and scrap sculpture workshops. Make the most of those that are enthusiastic and ask them to spread the word and chat to their neighbours about the initiative.

2. As with community allotment gardening (see Chapter 4), be clear from the outset what the intentions are for the project, how decisions are to be made, etc.

3. As coordinators of a community garden project, try to maintain a regular presence and make sure you are easily contactable by potential volunteers.

4. Coordination is a role that can benefit from being shared – it can be a lot for one person to take on, especially in a voluntary capacity.

5. Engage with local authorities, and housing/estate managers where relevant, as they can be an important source of support for the project and can help to generate local interest.

6. Harness the skills of community volunteers – there may be experienced events organisers, expert jam-makers, prize-carrot growers or PR gurus in your midst!

7. Keep up strong links with the wider Transition group and other relevant organisations in the area, attending meetings and events. News of your project will then be communicated back to other Transition folk who can use the site as a resource for developing their own gardening skills, meeting others and enjoying good food.

8. Hold facilitated work sessions, rather than leaving the site constantly open and often unattended.

9. Keep up the encouragement and compliments to new growers, and inspire them to grow their own at home by sharing cuttings, seeds and growing tips with them.

Resources

See page 192 for Community gardens, page 200 for General edible gardening, page 209 (More sources of help and interest) for permaculture resources, and page 197 for Funding, grants and loans.

Chapter 7
COMMUNITY ORCHARDS

If You Ate A Different Variety of Apple Everyday for Six Years You Wouldn't Have Tasted All The Varieties We Grow In Britain. 2,300 different Varieties of Dessert And Cooking Apple Have Been Grown Here.

Apple Day celebrations in Dunbar.
Photograph: Sustaining Dunbar

The UK currently imports 90 per cent of its fruit,[1] a statistic that stands in stark contrast to the rich heritage of orchards and fruit farms that once existed in Britain. The sad loss of these orchards has happened relatively recently – since the 1960s, the county of Wiltshire has lost 95 per cent of its traditional orchards, Devon has lost 90 per cent and Kent over 80 per cent.[2] As the land has been used for development of one kind or another, this country's ability to produce its own apples, plums and pears – rather than importing those from New Zealand and South Africa – has been drastically dented.

Orchards are not only a source of healthy, fresh fruit. They are also important places for wildlife; for perpetuating the growth of local fruit varieties and the traditions of juice- perry- and cider-making that accompany them; for spreading an appreciation of locally grown fruit; and as places of beauty, learning and enjoyment for the people that use them. For all these reasons, together with the looming threat of food insecurity, there has of late been a push to preserve those traditional orchards that still exist, and to establish new ones. The organisation Common Ground has been at the forefront of this movement, campaigning against the demolition of orchard sites, producing many publications in support of those that still exist, and initiating an annual celebration of the British apple, known as Apple Day, held in orchards across the country on 21 October. On this day, thousands of people attend events in their local orchards that include activities such as apple pressing, grafting and pruning workshops, orchard tours, and music, dancing and wassailing under the trees. Turning existing and privately owned orchards into community-run projects and establishing new community orchards are both encouraged by Common Ground as effective ways of allowing more people to enjoy and support orchards around the country.

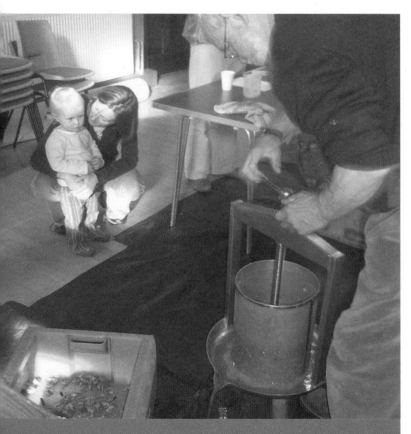

Preparing the apple press in front of a captivated audience at Sustaining Dunbar's Apple Day celebration. Photograph: Sustaining Dunbar

There are a number of practicalities that groups have to consider when going about setting up a community orchard. If taking over existing orchards, many of these sites will be made up of the larger, 'standard' trees that were traditionally planted in apple orchards in the UK. The height of these trees leaves them better protected from the animals that would also graze on the site. But in the community orchard setting, larger trees can pose problems for picking, as the fruit isn't easily accessible for harvest volunteers and the use of tall ladders can be potentially hazardous. Groups taking on the maintenance of these larger, established trees must therefore come up with other safe and practical ways of collecting and using their fruit. Choosing to make cider from the apples, for example, means that the fruit can be collected from the ground and ladder perils are avoided. But for groups planning and planting up new orchards, smaller trees can be a wiser, easier option.[3] There is then the issue of protecting these trees from grazing animals, unless the group chooses to tend or use the orchard grounds some other way (such as following the forest garden approach of growing edible shrubs, bushes and plants around the trees, as described on page 99).

Some of the above issues and suggestions apply only to orchards that are located on one specific site, as was traditionally always the case. But, as we shall see, there are other creative approaches to building a community orchard that are springing up within the local food movement, and that aren't dependent on finding one single site for the project.

Once a community orchard, in whatever form, is established, there are endless ways it can be used and enjoyed by local residents. Beyond the ideas described in this chapter (and depending on the specific site), they can also provide space for community cafes and celebrations, as well as for the growing of other fruit and vegetables and for beehives. Produce can be turned into juice, cider, perry, honey, jams, jellies, chutneys, cakes, biscuits and dried fruit that could be shared or sold to help support the orchard or other local initiatives. The timber from fruit trees is also a valuable resource, and mistletoe, which thrives in some orchards, can be picked and used as tinctures or for Christmas decorations.

On the following pages are the stories of three community orchard projects: one that has reclaimed and restored a traditional orchard, another that has established a new orchard site, and another that reinterprets the traditional definition of an 'orchard' by applying it to public spaces across an entire city.

Apples fresh from the tree. Photograph: Broadlands Community Orchard

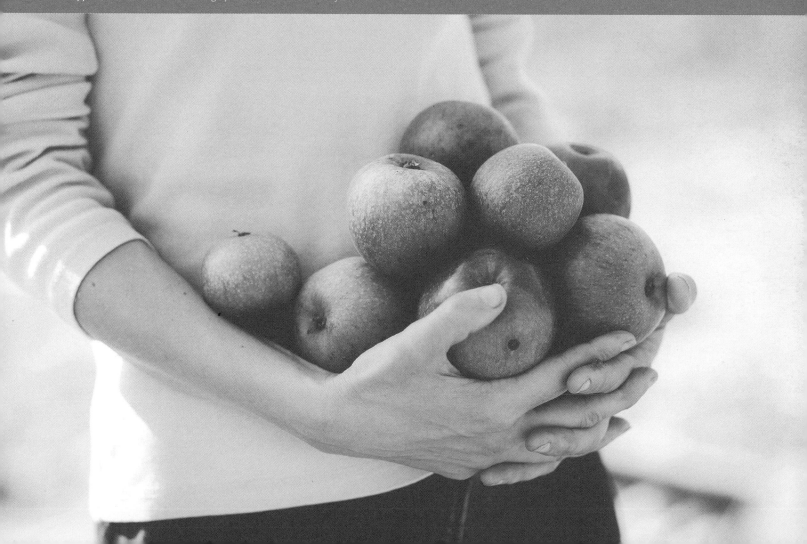

Community orchards – linking people, place and nature

Sue Clifford

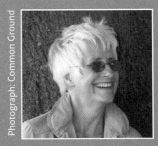

Photograph: Common Ground

In a community orchard of tall trees we can have it all: food for us and for myriad creatures, closeness to wild things, and connection with the land – the foundations of building a wiser life with nature.

Fruit trees have the advantage of growing very well on their own for most of the time, but when work is needed we can do much socially, learning from each other about aspect and slope, soil and season, variety and use. Doing things together makes it easy to pick up tips about pruning, grafting, storing, making juices and cider, creating tools and presses. Knowledge of local recipes, varieties of fruit particular to the place, new ideas can all be exchanged.

Orchards offer the richness of playground and pleasure garden, meeting place and festive stage. Rediscovering and inventing stories, songs, games and customs – ranging from wassailing to apple ducking – add layers of local distinctiveness, and rebuild community. And beauty comes free, poetry grows when nature and culture can rub along together. Climate change is but one symptom of our estrangement from where we live. We need to revalue our relations with nature in the deepest philosophical sense as well as very practically in our everyday surroundings. The community orchard compounds the power of the orchard as a working messenger of possibility and hope. Creating or conserving an orchard together can etch a philosophy of living well with the world, with culture and nature intertwining so well that there is room for both and richness in each.

Common Ground encourages people to actively create a new relationship with nature, starting in their own place – orchards across gardens holding the suburbs together, orchards at the heart of the village, fruit trees in smallholdings colonising the green belt, espaliered trees threading their way along walls in the city, roofs sprouting with coppiced nut trees, city fig and apricot gardens, fruit corners in parks, around workplaces, linear orchards along railways and canals, wild fruit in hedgerows – orchards linking town and country, place with place, people with nature.

Sue Clifford (together with Angela King) is a director of the organisation Common Ground, which works to link art and culture with the natural environment (see www.commonground.org.uk and Community orchards on page 193 of the Resources section for details of some of its publications).

Community orchard stories

Project name: Broadlands Community Orchard

Location: Bathford, Bath, UK

Aim: To engage local community in fruit growing and the importance of local food.

When established: 2006

How many people involved: 125 tree sponsors, up to twenty-five regular volunteers.

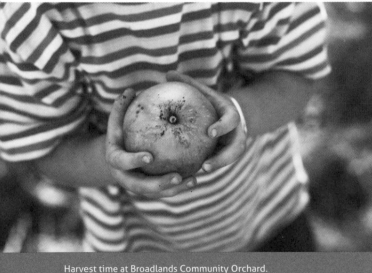

Harvest time at Broadlands Community Orchard.
Photograph: Graham Morgan photography

The idea

An example of a former commercial orchard that has been turned into a community resource valued by local residents is found in the village of Bathford, just outside the city of Bath. Here, the Broadlands Community Orchard has been operating since 2006, when the private owner agreed to grant the community access to the orchard rent-free, in return for 25 per cent of the annual harvest. Tim Baines, who is an experienced community gardener and who also works with the Federation of City Farms and Community Gardens (FCFCG), took on the role of coordinating the orchard because it was "too good an opportunity to miss" and because he thought it would provide an ideal way of demonstrating the importance of local food to people in the area.

The action

Tim and other volunteers are in the gradual process of restoring the mature, 11-acre orchard from a bramble jungle to its former prolific glory, and each year they expand their work to prune more of the 1,100 trees on the site. As well as providing an outdoor classroom for courses, workshops and workdays, the site is also a setting for regular events including, of course, Apple Day, and a traditional winter event complete with music from the local choir, tree decoration and a lamplit orchard tour. Tim has promoted the orchard and its produce at the Bath Farmers' Market (see page 115) as well as outside local shops, running an apple-pressing stall with apple bobbing for kids and free samples of juice for all.

To help fund the maintenance of the site, Tim and others have set up a tree sponsorship scheme whereby local residents pay £10 a year for the upkeep of their personally chosen tree (or up to five trees). Sponsors get to enjoy a box of their trees' apples, which they can collect from beneath the trees at harvest time. At the time of writing, just under 200 of the trees are sponsored – which, considering that the scheme's popularity has spread mainly by word of mouth, is a sure indication that the site is appreciated by local people.

As is the case with many community projects, Tim thinks that Broadlands could do with more volunteer input, but he is optimistic that people will be much more willing to offer their time and effort when there is less food in the shops!

Transition City Bath is fortunate to have the Broadlands Community Orchard in its locality and it supports and engages with the project – asking Tim to give presentations at meetings and promoting orchard events and activities through its network. Tim has noticed a rapid spread of awareness around Transition and local food in the area in recent months, with one development being the offer of 2 acres of land from the University of Bath to maintain an existing orchard and to develop a community food garden – a further example of how the existence of one community food project (such as the Broadlands Orchard) can inspire the emergence of others working towards the same, resilient ends.

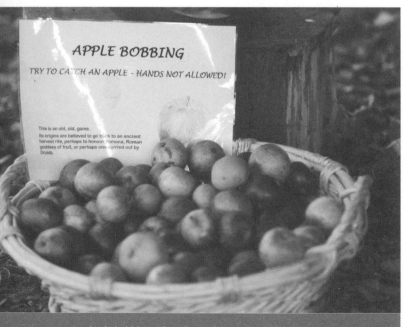

APPLE BOBBING

TRY TO CATCH AN APPLE - HANDS NOT ALLOWED!

This is an old, old, game.
Its origins are believed to go back to an ancient harvest rite, perhaps to honour Pomona, Roman goddess of fruit, or perhaps one carried out by Druids.

Apple bobbing at Broadlands Community Orchard.
Photograph: Graham Morgan photography

Project name: Donkey Field Community Orchard

Location: Portobello, Edinburgh, Scotland

Aim: To create a community orchard and inspire an appreciation of local food.

Started: September 2007

How many people involved: Thirty to forty

On the web: http://pedal-porty.org.uk/food/orchard

The idea

Further north, in Scotland, another community group has the related but different task of establishing a new orchard on a council-owned site in an urban area. The community-run environmental group PEDAL (Portobello Energy Descent and Land Reform Group) formed in Portobello, Edinburgh in 2005, and, inspired by the work of Transition Town Kinsale, decided to become the official Portobello Transition group in September 2007. Although its community orchard project is in the early stages, it has already attracted a lot of interest and support from local residents keen to get involved. Eva Schonveld, who helps to run the PEDAL group, has been pleasantly surprised by this reaction – of all the sustainability-related projects she has been involved in, it is the idea of a community orchard that has really grabbed people's imaginations.

PEDAL participants came up with the plans for the orchard when trying to think of locally engaged ways of feeding their community. They began by approaching the local council with the idea and a few suggestions of possible sites for the project. All were rejected, but others were offered and one, known as the Donkey Field, was eventually chosen. Although the site is further out of Portobello than the PEDAL group had hoped, it is situated among neighbourhoods that the group is keen to reach out to and gather interest from.

The action

Work on the Donkey Field Community Orchard was delayed while the council took some time to work out the terms of the lease – a source of frustration for those eager to get planting. But the council officer the group deals with is very supportive of the project, and now that the rent has been agreed, the 25-year lease settled and the papers signed, PEDAL is getting to work. At the time of writing, the first community planting session is getting under way, and the young fruit trees and bushes are going into the ground.

Eva and others were dealt a blow on the funding front when a grant application wasn't successful. Instead, the group members have had to come up with their own ways of raising funds (by holding two local food stalls in the town, and by selling sponsorship of the trees) to cover the annual £150 rent of the site and other project costs. Not receiving the grant has meant they have had to scale down their original vision for the time being, but they are hopeful that they will get the funds they need in the future and, in the meantime, their fundraising activities have had the added bonus of helping to boost the project's profile in the community.

The council has cleared the site for the project and has chipped existing sycamores, which will be used for paths and mulch. Planting has begun, and altogether the group will plant thirty fruit trees (focusing on the traditional and local varieties). Berry bushes, a willow plantation and a medicinal herb garden will also be added, and members are discussing the possibility of keeping bees on the site as well. In order to draw the community into the site, they will engage with local schools, run workshops and courses for local residents, and put up signs around the outside of the site to tell passers-by about the project's principles and aims. Fruit will be freely available for community members, and a group of PEDAL volunteers will oversee the planting, maintenance and harvest of the site. Non-local onlookers can keep an eye on the website for updates of the project's progress.

Project name: The Open Orchard Project
Location: Nelson, New Zealand
Aim: To plant, tend and harvest edible trees in public spaces around the city.
When established: February 2008
How many people involved: Over forty
Transition initiative website: www.transitionnelson.org.nz

The idea

The group in Portobello has been fortunate to find land for its orchard on city turf, but trying to establish new community orchards in land-scarce areas (common to many cities) isn't always possible. However, Nick Kiddey, a qualified arborist from the Transition City Nelson group in New Zealand, has found a way of turning this particular urban problem into an abundant opportunity. Having been inspired by similar initiatives in Southland and Wanganui, Nick decided to set up the Open Orchard project to plant native fruit and nut trees in existing public spaces around the city (such as parks, schools and in hospital grounds). He shared the idea with fellow Transitioners and, in February 2008, a group was formed dedicated to putting the plan into action.

The action

The Open Orchard was promoted in the press and on the radio, and was soon given the backing by the local council (as part of its healthy eating campaign), who agreed to provide $4,000 to purchase trees for planting.

More than forty people have already participated in the project, though Nick would like more volunteer input and is working on recruiting extra hands from the Nelson community. So far, activities have included mapping established and young edible trees in the city, educating volunteers on how to pick, prune and preserve, and producing a guide on 'what to plant where' for people inspired to plant their own trees at home. Nick points out that showing people what to do with the fruit once it has been grown is an essential part of the project's work, as there are many existing trees whose harvests have been wasted because of ignorance or a lack of interest.

Part of Open Orchard's approach is to try to share its idea with others – it is by no means a branded project protected by copyrights! – and to encourage more people to take it upon themselves to identify public spaces, seek permission and plant up some productive, native trees. It is Nick's hope that more people will be able to say, as he does, that "the city is my orchard". There are in fact many other villages, towns and cities that are already open orchards worldwide. Finding them is partly about opening our eyes to the wealth of edible trees, bushes and plants that already exist in rural and urban public spaces, but also about planting many more.

Some closing thoughts on community orchards

Community orchard projects come in many shapes and sizes. Transition Town Totnes's project to turn the town into a 'nut capital' is a further example of work that brings some edible inspiration to public lawns. And, by buying fruit trees in bulk and selling them at discounted prices for locals, Transition City Bristol's Virtual Orchard Initiative has encouraged more people to plant fruit trees in their own back gardens (as described by Claire Milne on page 182). All of these projects, and the enthusiasm generated around them, are helping to make more people see lawns and uncultivated spaces – whether public or private – as potential homes for edible trees.

Tips on setting up community orchards

As suggested by Tim Baines (Broadlands Community Orchard), Eva Schonveld (Donkey Field Community Orchard), Nick Kiddey (Open Orchard Project) and Frank Hemming (an orchard manager from Hereford-shire).

1. As Tim Baines says, "Go for it". Community orchards can be relatively easy projects to set up, with low capital input. They can even be done on small plots of land, with twenty sponsored trees and a couple of volunteers, or, with the council's backing, in public parks and spaces. Tim also thinks it's possible to learn as you go with new orchards, so don't let a lack of experience deter you.

Edible tree planting in a changing climate

Martin Crawford

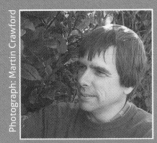

Photograph: Martin Crawford

Growing annual food crops uses lots of energy – you can't get away from that fact. If not fossil-fuel energy then it will be animal and/or human energy. But tree crops (and other perennial crops) don't need so much energy to cultivate. You plant them only once, they need little tending, just a bit or pruning and mulching, and just require harvesting. There are varieties of most fruit and nut trees suited to almost any region or location, so with sensible choices you can productive trees that are disease-resistant wherever you are.

In the face of climate change not all varieties of, for example, apple trees will continue to thrive well in their indigenous homelands. They may well be good varieties and some will adapt to changing conditions better than others, but gradually their optimum locations are moving northwards as climate zones shift. So Devon apples will soon be of more value in Wales, whilst apples from north-west France will be valuable in Devon.

A forest garden is a kind of underplanted orchard – you start with fruit and nut trees, and with careful design and placement, shrub crops and perennials are grown beneath – all can be useful edible plants, though you can't really grow the 'normal' annual vegetables in shade. Forest gardens are more than this, though – they are aesthetically beautiful places, which can reconnect people with nature in the same way that a wild forest can do.

Martin Crawford is a forest gardener, teacher, director of the Agroforestry Research Trust and author of Agroforestry Options for Landowners *(see his website, www. agroforestry.co.uk, for details on further agroforestry publications and resources). He and his forest garden are featured on the DVD* A Forest Garden Year.

2. Be aware that when working with volunteers in the orchard, it is inevitable that some mistakes will occur – there is only so much people can learn about pruning in an introductory session. But (assuming they are committed in the long term) their skills will improve over time. In the meantime, do what you can to ensure there aren't any severe casualties (to person or tree)!

3. Establish good and regular communication with the local council, whether you decide to lease a site from it or not, as having it on side can be useful for supporting and potentially promoting your project.

4. Have people on the team (or at least in touch with the team) who are experienced orchard growers; they are invaluable as a source of insight and information.

5. Make sure your workload is sufficiently covered by core group members – often, new volunteers are more keen to get involved with the planting than the planning side of things.

6. Remember that a lack of funding can be disappointing but it just means the group will have to come up with (potentially more fun) ways of raising money.

7. Have a good think about health and safety issues (especially where ladders are concerned), as there are tales of orchard activities that have gone horribly wrong – which leads to the following tip . . .

8. Be sure to take out insurance on the project to cover any mishaps that may occur.

9. Sign up to Martin Crawford's newsletter (see www.agroforestry.co.uk) – a very helpful source of information, including details of which trees are resistant to which diseases.

10. It might be worth securing a space to store fruit in case you have a glut you're unable to share out or sell. One tried-and-tested method for storing apples is to leave them out in the sun to sweat (if warm enough), then to store them four or five apples deep in a dry space at about 4°C, making sure to check them each week for rotting.

11. Plant new orchard projects with smaller trees that have low-hanging fruit, and if the group does choose to have animals grazing on the site, remember that sheep are easier by far to manage than cattle. Picking practicalities are just some of the considerations to be aware of when choosing trees for a new community orchard – see below for more.

12. Choose trees that are suited to the climate and soil of the orchard site.

13. Favour popular fruit varieties that local residents will like, perhaps consulting them on the choices beforehand.

14. Ensure you have a good range of trees (including different fruit and nut varieties).

15. Plant those that will not require too much maintenance (trees that are described as 'requiring careful cultivation' will most likely need much attention and hard work and are therefore unlikely to be a good choice for a community orchard).

Resources

See page 193 for Community orchards and page 197 for Funding, grants and loans.

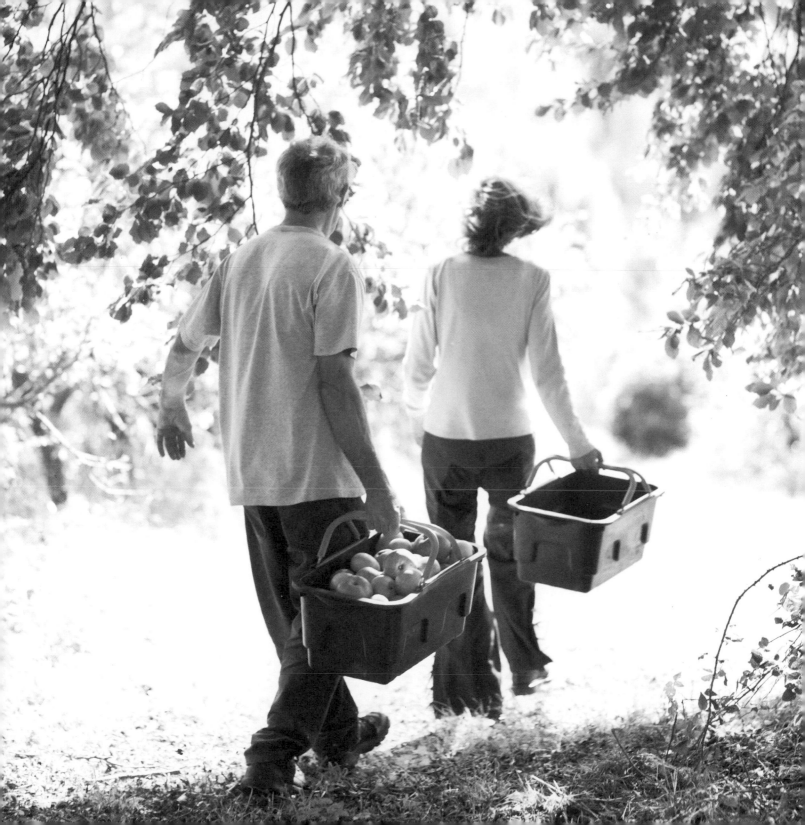

Chapter 8
COMMUNITY SUPPORTED AGRICULTURE

In the UK and around the world, Community Supported Agriculture schemes (often referred to as CSAs) are fast becoming recognised as key elements of local food networks, and as efficient, resilient ways of feeding communities. CSAs come in many shapes and sizes but they are in essence farms (often set up as limited companies) in which community members become involved by buying shares, making decisions and even helping to grow and harvest the food they eat.

Setting up a CSA can be a larger project than those described in other chapters in this book, requiring much groundwork, knowledge and community support before it can take off. But because the CSA model strengthens relationships between the farmer, the community and the wider environment, there are many benefits that come with the start-up and long-term effort it requires. For the farmers, there is a secure market for the food they produce. For the community members that support them, there is access to local, often organic food, the opportunity to develop their own growing skills and the space to have a say in what is produced and how. Because the food producers are growing for a defined, local market rather than for the unpredictable, global food market, the food miles that their produce travels are drastically reduced and they are able to support wildlife and biodiversity by growing a varied selection of crops. So although the term 'Community Supported Agriculture' implies a one-way relationship of support from the community to the farmer, the relationships are actually three-way (between growers, community and the environment) and the benefits flow in all directions. Gaps between the three recipients are closed, understanding is fostered, and each receives the nourishment it deserves (see Amanda Daniel's article on page 105 for the Soil Association's views on why CSAs have an important role to play in local food networks). Because CSAs prioritise ethics over profit they can be described as a type of social enterprise. This means that even if they choose to operate as profit-making businesses, any surplus that is made is put back into the initiative to help further its community- and environment-focused aims.

The CSA approach to farming first emerged in the 1960s as an early reaction to the increased industrialisation of agriculture and the stretching of food supply chains. As a way of bringing farming back in touch with the communities it feeds, groups in Germany, Switzerland and Japan began setting up direct and supportive relationships with local farmers to source their own fresh, safe food. In Japan, this model is known as *teikei,* which translates as 'putting the farmer's face on the food' – an apt description for a model that narrows the otherwise ubiquitous consumer–producer divide.

In the 1980s CSA schemes spread to the USA, where they have since grown to include more than 1,500 farms and surrounding communities. In the UK their uptake has been slower, but recently the numbers of CSAs have steadily increased to over 100. Because the model effectively addresses the pressing issues of rising food prices, environmental damage and community disconnection from farming, it is likely that more and more CSAs will spring up in this country in coming years.

While CSA is a loose and growing category that has come to encompass a whole range of farmer–community linked schemes (including subscription box schemes and cooperatives made up of two or more farms), many of them can be said to share the following core principles.

- There is an agreement of shared risk between the farmers and the consumers, so that the CSA has shareholder support (and monthly shares are paid) whether or not crops fail or yields are low. This means that the farmer's security of income is based upon an agreed trust with the community, rather than on the vagaries of the markets or the unpredictability of the weather.

- Many CSAs emphasise the importance of transparency in the way the farm is organised and in the relationship between farmer and community shareholders. Ways of maintaining transparency include democratic or consensus-based decision-making amongst members, elected management committees, weekly opportunities for shareholders to help and learn on the farm, regular open meetings and good communication channels between everyone involved. One benefit of encouraging high levels of trust between those that grow the food and those that eat it is that, since many CSAs adhere strictly to organic or biodynamic principles anyway, the sometimes-costly process of organic certification is not necessary. If, on the other hand, the CSA wants to sell surplus produce to the local market under the label 'organic', or if members choose to have the security of independent, organic verification, then it may benefit from certification and the technical support that comes with it.

- CSAs are designed to be financially beneficial to all involved, as well as to the community at large. The farmers generally receive a higher and more secure income than those that grow and sell to an external market. Because of the low overheads (through limited use of packaging and transport), CSA-produced food is often cheaper than similar non-organic produce from supermarkets. Research undertaken by members of Stroud Community Agriculture found, for example, that the price of their vegetable share (£7.38) was lower than that of the same produce from Tesco, Waitrose, Sainsbury's or the Co-op.[1] In a wider sense, CSAs contribute to a strengthening of the local economy by making sure that money spent on food stays in the community and helps to support a locally based food initiative.

- Lastly, and for some reasons already mentioned, CSAs support and promote community resilience. By involving farms that are locally situated and organic, CSAs are an efficient way of feeding communities in a post-fossil-fuel era. A good diversity of crops and/or livestock means that a community can remain well fed even if one crop fails. And, because of the strong farmer–community bonds that it relies upon, it helps to promote community cohesion and cooperation, and to value the farmer's role (and the production of local, organic food in general) within the community.

There are CSA rumblings happening in urban and rural communities all across the Transition Network, including those springing from Transition initiatives in Bristol, Falmouth, Exeter and Kinsale. Many of these are in their visioning and planning stages, and it will be exciting to see what transformative effects they have on the communities they feed and engage with. There follow two examples of shareholder CSAs in the UK that are already up and running, and that are born of or linked with their local Transition groups. The first is well established and has been going for eight years, and we shall look at this in some detail. The second is newer and smaller (and the description of it is more brief), but the differences between them help to illustrate the various shapes that CSAs fill, and to show how the CSA approach allows projects to be moulded by the people, place and principles that they are a part of.

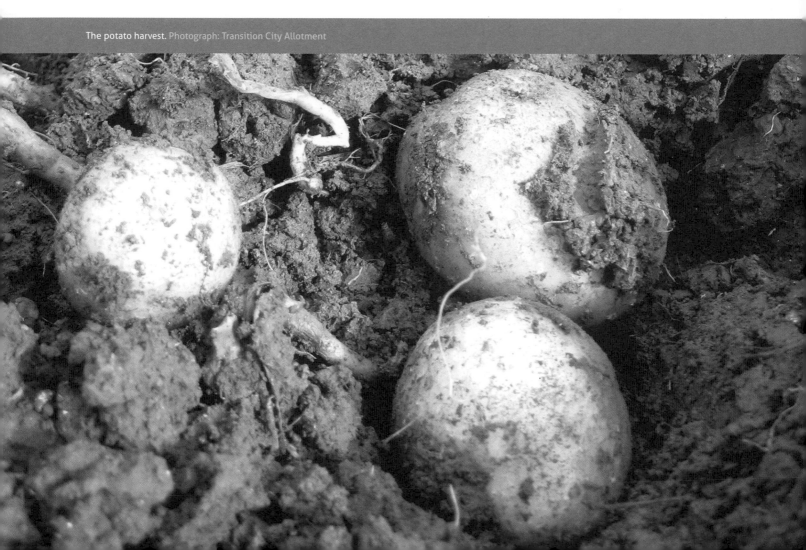

The potato harvest. Photograph: Transition City Allotment

An alternative food future

Amanda Daniel

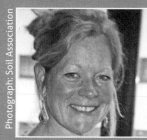

Photograph: Soil Association

There are now dozens of Community Supported Agriculture (CSA) schemes emerging throughout the UK. The Soil Association is both supporting communities and farmers in the development of many of these and investigating the potential role of CSAs in an energy-lean future. CSA schemes offer a practical response to the food challenges that face us, through their capacity to create localised, lower-carbon food production and trading systems, based on mutually beneficial partnerships between food producers and surrounding communities.

Sustainable production

As CSA commonly uses organic farming and growing methods, a means of food production that avoids the use of pesticides and prohibits synthetic fertilisers, the reliance on fossil fuels is reduced. Dependence on mechanised methods of production is also lessened, as, in some examples, volunteer work days give members the opportunity to become directly involved in the CSA. With members collecting their share of fresh produce directly from the farm shortly after harvesting, the need for facilities such as plastic packaging, cold storage and extensive distribution can be removed.

Committed customers and a secure income

Through CSA, a very different connection between the farmer and 'consumer' is being created, based on commitment and trust. CSA establishes a customer base that ensures the farmer receives a fair price, which is paid in advance. This offers an economically viable model of food production to the farmer, enabling him or her to establish a more sustainable business in the long term. The members' 'share' price is set at the start of the season and price increases tend to be minimal, as the farm is less dependent on external markets. This allows farmers to budget in advance for their business and members for their living expenses.

Reskilling communities

Being involved with a CSA scheme is enabling people to connect with the land from which their food is produced. This is creating numerous opportunities to develop new skills and learn how to produce food. Working together as a community to establish a CSA scheme means sharing ideas and skills to jointly create positive change.

An adaptable approach

CSAs can be established in rural areas or in urban settings, on municipal land, farms, allotments or gardens. The initial motivation can come either from farmers or from local people. Through thinking creatively about the opportunities that available land provides, and creating connections with centres of population, CSAs provide an opportunity to restructure food production, marketing and distribution.

Sustainable food plan for Britain

The principles of the CSA approach underpin the Soil Association's 'manifesto for action' that supports our sustainable food plan for Britain. We believe that a radical transformation of farming methods and the reconstruction of more localised food processing and distribution networks is vital, in order to rebuild food and farming communities, support low-carbon farming and empower and engage individuals.

Amanda Daniel is the Information Officer for the Soil Association's CSA team (see www.soilassociation.org/csa and www.makinglocalfoodwork.co.uk for more information).

CSA stories

Project name: Stroud Community Agriculture (SCA)

Location: Stroud, Gloucestershire

Aim: To provide local, organic food for local people, encourage mutual cooperation between farmers and consumers, and reduce the community's dependence on fossil-fuelled food.

Started: 2001

How many people involved: Four paid farmers, one paid administrator/treasurer, and nearly 200 members, of whom nine are elected to sit on the management group.

On the web: www.stroudcommunityagriculture.org

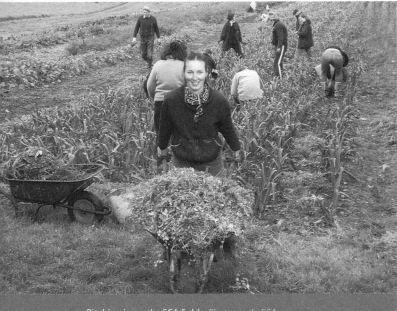

Pitching in on the SCA fields. Photograph: SCA

The idea

The Stroud Community Agriculture scheme (SCA) was one of the first and most productive CSAs to have started up in the UK, and it has since gone on to support and inspire a number of newer CSA initiatives around the country. In 2001 a group of four Stroud residents got together to discuss ways of supporting food resilience in their area and of providing local, organic food for their families. The plan they came up with was to try to start a CSA on the site of a local farm that was going through a hard patch and that would benefit from community support. The first step was to hold a public meeting about the idea so that they could gauge opinion and see whether the scheme would have community backing. The group got in touch with Jade Bashford and others at the Soil Association, who helped plan a presentation about why there was a need for a CSA in Stroud, and a local farmer was invited to come and discuss the struggles that small farms can face in the UK. Time was put aside for free discussion at the end of the meeting, and posters were put up around the hall where people could write down their own ideas for the CSA, offer their services or be put on a mailing list. The meeting was a resounding success, with over eighty people attending and much support being given to the plan – so the group decided to go ahead.

Although SCA was established with a wide ownership base of community shareholders, it was, in the beginning, officially run by the core group as an unincorporated association. This meant that it was the core group members who would be held legally responsible if anything went wrong (such as injuries occurring on the farm). Further down the line, and in order to spread the burden of responsibility more evenly, SCA was set up as an industrial and provident society in 2002. Principles of democratic decision-

have access to local, organic food by working part-time at the farm to pay for some of their share. Most members pick up their vegetables from the packing shed on the SCA farm, where a blackboard lists the quantities of vegetables assigned to each share and the SCA member weighs them up and boxes them him- or herself. Members can also buy cheese, eggs or meat there, registering their purchase by leaving payment in the honesty box. Alternatively, members can pick their shares up from two collection points in Stroud.

Nick Weir is one of the original core group members of SCA and still supports and is involved in the initiative. According to Nick, a flat, open structure is fundamental to community-engaged food production, and at SCA there are a number of different ways its members have access to decision-making within the project. For instance, the farmers decide what to grow based on responses to share-holder questionnaires and suggestions from the open meetings that are held regularly. SCA also holds an annual harvest supper and a conversation cafe (where views and suggestions are written on paper tablecloths and collected by core group members) – all opportunities to help shape the project. If someone has a particularly burning issue to air, he or she is always welcome to attend core group sessions too. Shareholders can also elect new core group members at AGMs (the core group now being made up of up to nine people), and, together with SCA's farmers, the core group then makes decisions affecting the direction and running of the project.

Nick points out that although roughly 70 per cent of the shareholders choose not to contribute to decision-making and are happy just to collect their vegetables, chat with the farmer and occasionally work on the farm, having the mechanisms in place that allow access to the running of the project creates a greater sense of ownership, trust and commitment among members. And, crucially, if anyone in the initiative (from the consumers to the producers) doesn't like what's happening, they can do something about it – an approach that signifies a radical departure from the top-down decision-making strategies and frequently harmful policies of the supermarkets.

Beyond decision-making, there are numerous ways shareholders can get involved with the project, including joining sub-groups (such as the festivals group that helps organise various events), working voluntarily on the farm, attending festivals, dinners, bonfires and camping weekends held at the site and taking part in the August haymaking. Should they so wish, they are even invited to partake in an alternative carol concert on Christmas Eve, to an audience of CSA cows.

The core group itself is run by consensus, which, according to Nick, requires much trust, clear communication, and the letting-go of personal ideals for all involved. It is a process that can be anything from painful to beautiful, but that eventually gives rise to strongly determined, intelligent decisions, and that is agreed to be deeply rewarding overall.

Beyond SCA

As mentioned in Chapter 4, the town of Stroud has a thriving Transition group that has linked up with existing local food initiatives, and there are a number of SCA members who are also active in Transition. Some people have found out about SCA via the Transition group (and vice versa), and Nick points out that Transition Town Stroud is an important forum through which to promote SCA as a local, successful example of community engagement through food production. SCA members have recently begun exploring ways of making their project less reliant on mains supplies and fossil fuels, by harvesting and using rainwater and by replacing some of the tractor work with working horses.

Keen to share their experiences and lessons learnt with other fledgling CSAs, SCA members have participated in a number of talks, workshops and conferences, as well as hosting reporters from various TV and radio programmes. The thinking behind this willingness to share SCA's story comes from a conviction that the project isn't just about feeding Stroud but about being part of a wider move towards food resilience, in which good practice, visions and ideas are within easy common reach.

Project name: Canalside Community Food

Location: Near Leamington Spa, Warwickshire

Aim: To provide local, seasonal, organic produce with and for the community.

Started: 2006

How many people involved: Three growers, one administrator, seven steering group members and 110 shareholders.

On the web: www.canalsidecommunityfood.org.uk

The idea

One CSA that drew inspiration and support from the folk in Stroud is the Canalside Community Food initiative in Warwickshire. In comparison with SCA, this project is at an earlier stage in its formation and has grown from a differing set of circumstances. Tom and Caz Ingall had been excited about the idea of setting up a CSA for a few years before they decided to take the plunge and turn their words into actions. In 2005 they managed to persuade Tom's parents to let them use some of their farmland for CSA food production (which they soon started to convert to organic), and were then in the position of having land for the project, but no grower. This is in contrast to many projects that often find it easier to come by growers than they do land. Through local connections the Ingalls soon established a steering group of seven committed members who could take the project to the wider community – posts that would be re-elected by CSA members at each future AGM. They were also able to find someone prepared to be the grower for the project, so all they then needed was the community support to get things going.

Unlike the town of Stroud, where a local, organic food market is popular and visible, Tom and Caz live in an area where, according to them, an awareness of local food issues is yet to appear on the radar. So they were

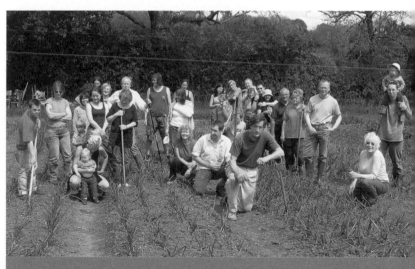

Many hands make happier, lighter work at a Canalside Community work day.
Photograph: Canalside Community Food CSA

thrilled (and a little frightened) when, having delivered and handed out 5,000 leaflets describing the idea and inviting community input, over ninety local residents turned up to their first public meeting. A number of people signed up to the project there and then, but the quickly formed steering group made the decision that it was a lot to ask new members to pay up front before any food was grown (as some did with SCA), and that they wanted responsibility to be more evenly spread among members. Instead, through sharing their idea with the community, the project was given the support of a generous local resident who came forward and gave them a loan of £10,000 to help get things going – a wonderful example of the 'sowing and reaping' theme described on page 30.

Many CSAs, like SCA on page 106, choose to provide their members with a wider range of fruit and vegetables by buying some produce in from other local farmers or by forging trade links with producers abroad. The Canalside team decided to take the less common route of supplying entirely fresh, local and seasonal produce grown on their farm. Tom, Caz and others chose to go down this path because they wanted the challenge of creating a market for the purely local. This means that their members may go about sourcing some non-local fruit and vegetables for themselves, especially in some of the 'hungrier' months, but it gives them the opportunity to enjoy what is locally seasonal as a starting point for their families' food, and to supplement it as suits them. This commitment to their own-grown food has led to some nerve-racking times at Canalside, but putting up five polytunnels has allowed them to extend their growing season and stick to their original principles.

Inspired by the work of Iain Tolhurst, an organic farmer from Berkshire who has pioneered animal-free, organic agriculture for over twenty years, they are now exploring ways to gradually reduce animal inputs by experimenting with green manures. They hope to provide an example of how a farm can still operate efficiently if it is stock-free – an approach that many farms may have to shift towards in a post-fossil-fuel future in order to maximise the efficiency of their land use.[2]

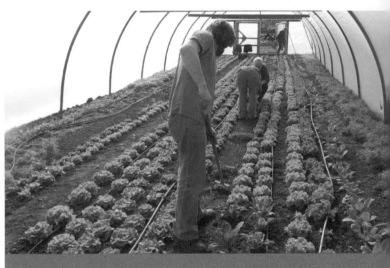

Inside the Canalside polytunnel.
Photograph: Canalside Community Food CSA

The action

When they started out Tom and Caz had experience of vegetable gardening but not of field-scale growing. They didn't, however, let this restrain their ambitious visions. Instead, Tom decided to do some volunteer work at the nearby site of the charity Garden Organic (see www.gardenorganic.co.uk) to build up his skills. There he got to know experienced local gardener Thalia Nunis, who later agreed to work for Canalside as a paid consultant, helping to plan their planting and crop rotations and work out what quantity of food would need to be grown for their projected number of CSA shares. The steering group decided to set the limit at ninety small shares in its first year, which, in February for example, might include 1.5kg of potatoes, 650g of carrots, 400g of onions, 1 small cabbage, 1 swede, 250g of purple sprouting broccoli and one mixed salad bag. They worked out that producing for ninety small shares would be enough to cover the wages and project running costs. This took into account their reliance on volunteer help and community input, with all members being encouraged to come and help on the farm at their open sessions on Wednesday and Saturday mornings. By the time of their first harvest, however, only forty-five small shares had been taken up, so they began selling the excess produce to local wholefood shops to make up the extra funds. But word of their tasty vegetables continued to spread, and by October they were on target, producing for ninety small shares. Eighty of these were paid for in full, and ten were given free to the growers or as part of work-share arrangements based on the SCA model described on pages 106-9.

At this point the Canalside team made the mistake of telling people that their membership list was full, without making it clear that it would not always be the case. This meant that when they later wanted to extend their share limit to 110, there was still the perception among local residents that there were no more available shares, and it took a good year to get the message back out that their was membership space on offer. Share numbers are now steadily on the increase again, and Tom estimates that the final share limit that their space will allow is approximately 140.

Canalside's nearest Transition initiative is Leamington Spa (TTLS), a group that decided to amend its constitution in order to include the CSA in its catchment area (as an important example of local, sustainable, community farming). Though there are not yet formal links between the two organisations, a few members of Canalside's steering group are also active in groups within the Transition initiative. Each is supportive of the other's work, and TTLS recently demonstrated this support by granting £500 from its main budget to fund the building of a straw-bale toilet block at the farm. At Canalside they are keenly aware of the need to make a move away from fossil-fuel dependence, and they try to do as much of their work as possible without the use of machinery. They have also been exploring a number of energy-efficient ideas such as heating covered growing spaces with their own coppiced willow, converting tractors to their own, farm-produced biodiesel and reducing the amount of carbon released from ploughing by increasing the number of perennial plants and edible trees they keep. Their hope is that, once they're beyond the 'keeping heads above water' stage, they'll have more time to focus on 'peak-oil-proofing' the project.

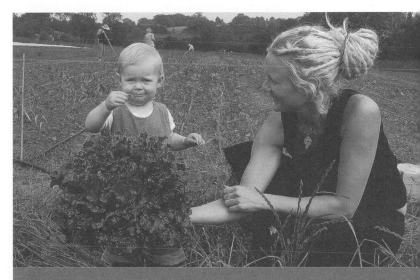

You're never too young to pick lettuce, even if it's nearly as big as you are.
Photograph: Canalside Community Food CSA

Some closing thoughts on CSAs

The projects mentioned in this chapter are examples of how, when communities engage with food production, they develop a passion for good food and a deep respect for the land that provides it, so that consequences for the local and global environment can be positive and far-reaching. From using working horses in Stroud to providing only organic, local produce at Canalside, CSAs find their own ways of working respectfully with the Earth, cutting agricultural pollution and preparing for a fossil-fuel-lean future. Once a CSA is established, its members can use the project as a vehicle for exploring and working through such ideas, while maintaining the productivity of their farm.

A powerful and common thread to many CSA stories (as mentioned previously), is that the community often delivers and provides what the project needs. When an initiative of this kind is put in the community domain it is opened up to a wider pool of skills, resources, labour, knowledge, funds, materials and even land. CSA founders are regularly amazed by what assistance comes their way when they ask for it. Further examples of this kind of community help include that enjoyed by the Farnham Local Food Initiative, which, on the back of a public meeting held in 2008, received four offers of land and much of the labour (given voluntarily) that it requires to operate (see www.farnhamfood.com for more information). And, on the recently established CSA in Hastings (set up by Transition City Hastings member Joel Brook), all of the growing is undertaken by local volunteers, who are honing their gardening skills while also providing food for their community. The kind of community engagement facilitated by CSAs generates and harnesses passionate enthusiasm among the people who participate in it, and this is due, in no small part, to the sheer thrill that comes from being able to shape and engage with the food system that feeds us.

Tips on setting up a CSA

As suggested by Nick Weir (SCA), Tom Ingall (Canalside Community Food CSA), Susie Tavare (Farnham Local Food Initiative CSA) and Joel Brook (Hastings CSA).

1. It is very important to open the CSA vision up to wider input and ownership as early as possible. It is much harder to try to sell an established vision to a community than it is to draw it into the visioning and creative process at the outset. The project will then have a wider ownership base and a larger pool of skills, minds and enthusiasm.

2. Try to resist the temptation to apply for funding too early on, before the project's identity and self-sufficiency have had a chance to form. This can stifle creativity and the autonomy of the project. Other ways of raising start-up funds that may have fewer strings attached include arranging a loan (from a private person, ethical bank or social investment fund), asking new members to pledge investments, or finding a local benefactor to support the project. See pages 197-9 for organisations that can help finance CSAs.

3. Visit other CSAs, talk to their members and take advantage of the help and support provided by the Soil Association (including reading its CSA Action Manual, downloadable from www.soilassociation.org/csa) and its CSA team (contact details in Resources section – see opposite).

4. It would be helpful, in the early days, for the core group or management committee to dig beneath the assumption that they all hold the same vision and to make differences clear and understood. This will prepare the ground for greater cooperation and smoother decision-making down the line.

5. Try not to get too caught up in the idea that you need an experienced grower in order to start up a CSA. According to Tom Ingall, if you have enough enthusiasm and if you pull in the services of a more knowledgeable person to be on call and to point you in the right direction, then the necessary learning will happen quickly. It is also important not to underestimate the usefulness of unskilled labour – volunteer help plays a large role at Canalside and gives members a chance to feel they're part of the project and the community around it.

6. Publicity can be very useful in raising the project's profile and recruiting support, and so it is a good idea to get local media on board at an early stage.

7. Cherish your volunteers and give them the time and attention they deserve! They will be much more likely to continue working with the project if they feel appreciated and part of it. Keep them informed of CSA news and meetings; give them the chance to develop their skills and learn new ones; hold regular, fun, social events on the site; and encourage them to share ideas and suggestions for the project.

8. Don't be put off by the lack of obvious 'deep green' sympathies in your area – establishing a CSA often manages to draw support from the most unlikely corners of a community, and can pull closet food lovers out of the woodwork.

9. Try to establish links with other local farms and food-growing projects, so that support, skills, tips and perhaps labour, machinery and land can be shared.

10. Use the project to help make sure local, organic food is accessible to everyone in the community. The CSA can be opened out to low-income members by operating a work-share scheme, instalment plans or a sliding scale of share prices, or by inviting other members or businesses to subsidise some of the shares.

Resources

See page 193 for CSAs and page 197 for Funding, grants and loans.

Chapter 9

FARMERS' MARKETS

A farmers' market is one where farmers sell their own produce directly to the consumers. They thereby pocket 80-90 per cent of the consumers' spending as opposed to the 8-10 per cent they might otherwise get selling to supermarkets and large-scale food distributors.[1] Once a central outlet for food produce and a regular hub of community activity, farmers' markets virtually disappeared across the industrialised world as imported food and national, centralised distribution networks came to dominate the food sector. But they took off again in the US in the 1980s, with numbers growing from 100 to 1,755 between 1976 and 1994,[2] and started to be re-established in the UK in the late 1990s. In more recent years the UK's National Farmers' Retail and Market Association (FARMA) has seen a sharp rise in its membership, from under 200 farmers' markets in 2000 to nearly 800 in 2009.

Farmers' markets vary in size, produce, popularity and principles, depending on their venue, the surrounding agricultural context, the teams that run them and the people that they sell to. FARMA has strict guidelines on what constitutes a verified farmers' market, and its members can pay to be certified in this way. All stallholders must sell only their own products (whether these are primary, such as vegetables and fruit, or secondary, such as bread and cakes), but the limit of what defines them as 'local producers' varies. The maximum distance producers can travel to a market if they are to be called 'local' (according to

FARMA) is 100 miles, but some farmers' markets limit the distance to 50 and even 30 miles. Farmers' markets within urban areas are often more lenient on the distances producers may travel, simply because they are held further away from agricultural land.

There are a number of markets that call themselves 'farmers' markets' and that actually allow stallholders to sell produce that is imported (or at least not local) or produced by someone other than the stallholder, so it is always worth finding out what a market's principles are before assuming it's the genuine article. Farmers' markets are also not to be confused with the many other types of market that are seen around the UK, such as permanent covered markets (where stallholders operate what are essentially small shops) or commercially run street markets (where there is often a large variety of products, from T-shirts to dog bowls, and little restriction on what is sold or where it comes from). Neither of these are ideal outlets for small food producers, who can benefit more from selling produce at a market specifically geared to their quality of produce and with the purpose of supporting local producers.

One other type of market that *is* popular with small producers is what was formerly known as the Women's Institute Market, and what is now called the Country Market (see www.country-markets.co.uk). Run as non-profit-making cooperatives all over the UK, there are at the time of writing over 400 of these markets attended by more than 12,000 small producers, many of whom make their products in their own homes. They first started in 1919, when the Agricultural Organisation Society (the government body now known as Defra) commissioned the Women's Institute (WI) to run cooperative markets as outlets for surplus agricultural products, and over the years they have steadily developed a reputation for selling high-quality jams, pickles, fruit, vegetables, cakes and breads. To be able to sell at an existing Country Market a producer must become a shareholder in the organisation (and it costs only 5p for one share), acquire a food hygiene safety certificate, give a small commission of its profits to the running of the market (usually between 10 and 15 per cent) and be prepared to help staff stalls and run the whole market alongside others. Because Country Markets Ltd offers training, advice and full product and public liability insurance to its producer members, this is a cheap, supportive way of selling home-made and/or home-grown produce. Country Markets' long, successful experience in organising food-selling events also leaves a lot of scope for groups wanting to set up farmers' markets in the same area, as forces can be joined and venues, skills and labour can be shared.

As well as opening up a space for producer–consumer connection, farmers' markets, once established, can become important places for community interaction – for showcasing entertainment from local artists and musicians, for the promotion of other community groups, campaigns and events, and as an opportunity to raise awareness of local food issues in general. Consumers are much more likely to consider the links between the environment, the welfare of farmers, the cost of food and their own nutrition if they have the opportunity to meet the people who produce their food, to talk about where it comes from and to think about how it is grown or made. Described below is a well-known and established project that has helped to reignite a national love of farmers' markets, followed by two that are newer and smaller in scale. All of them have a commitment to local food at their core, but that is manifested in different ways.

Farmers' market stories

Project name: Bath Farmers' Market

Location: Bath, Somerset

Aim: To set up a producer-managed market, run along principles of environmental sustainability, where small and new local producers can sell directly to consumers.

Started: 1997

How many people involved: One director, one manager, a management committee of seven, between twenty-five and thirty stallholders, and up to 5,000 customers at each market.

On the web: www.bathfarmersmarket.co.uk

The idea

Peter Andrews, a publisher from Bath, has been active in local food issues for many years and was part of the original team that set up the Bath Farmers' Market – the first of its kind in the whole of UK. The idea surfaced back in 1997 when Peter was chatting with one of his authors about the rise of farmers' markets in the US. He was grabbed by what he thought would be a sure way of promoting local food and creating an outlet for small-scale producers. So, together with contacts from local groups, he embarked on a mission to turn the idea into reality.

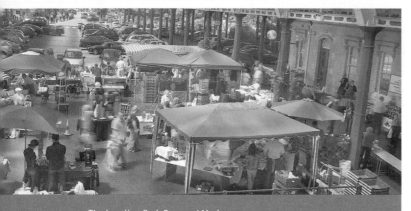

The bustling Bath Farmers' Market.
Photograph: Scott Morrison Photography

The action

A team of organisers was pulled together for the project, which included two people who worked for the local council, and a number of others experienced in small-scale food production, horticulture and permaculture. Having the council's backing was key to getting the market plans off the ground, as it helped to make a site at Green Park Station available at a relatively low cost, promoted the farmers' market, and provided the organising team with secretarial support. The organisers got in touch with local producers using the permaculture group's recently compiled local food directory (one example of the way such directories can be used as a resource for other local food projects – see Chapter 11 for more on guides and directories), and received a good response. Peter and others thought it important to make sure, from the beginning, that there was a good balance of producers on the stalls, allowing for some competition without boring consumers with an over-abundance of any one product.

On the first day, twenty-six producers took part, including local allotment growers, beekeepers and a group from the WI. The market was a resounding success, with about 3,000 people turning up, and some organic vegetables selling out by midday. Even the nearby shops benefited from the market's presence, as they drew in more custom from the increased numbers of passers-by. Peter took the project's popularity as evidence that the farmers' market's time had come – that consumers were ready and enthusiastic to start supporting their local producers once more – and it was decided, after a three-month trial, that it would continue as a weekly fixture on the same site. The story of the market's speedy success was picked up by many local and national radio and TV journalists and spread far and wide. Within a matter of months, other farmers' markets had sprung up all around the country and have continued to do so ever since.

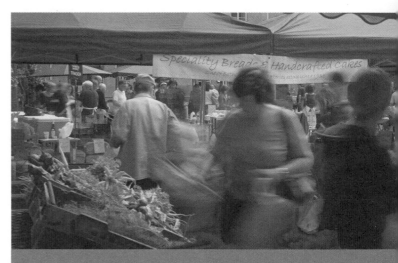

Happy shoppers at the Bath Farmers' Market.
Photograph: Scott Morrison Photography

The way it works

Peter and other organisers decided that they didn't want to be permanent market managers – they saw their role more as catalysts to get things started. Instead they set up a management committee that the stallholders took on and ran themselves, registering as a limited company in June of 1998. It was decided that in order to be a farmers' market stallholder, producers would become market members by paying an annual fee that would also entitle them to vote for positions in the management committee. Stallholders pay a weekly rental fee for their pitch (which at the time of writing is £20 each), and it is their responsibility to arrange hygiene certificates and public, employee and product liability insurance themselves.

Keith Goverd has been the market's director (as appointed by the management committee) for much of the time since the early days, and he points out that the system they operate is simple but effective. Any concerns that do arise among customers or stallholders are relayed back to Keith and dealt with as necessary – there is a reliance upon close, communicative relationships in the marketplace (from the shopper to the producer) to ensure that issues are aired and everyone is happy. According to Keith, things generally run smoothly and are issue-free.

Principles of local, sustainable agriculture were placed at the heart of the Bath Farmers' Market from the outset. For its organisers, this meant prioritising the small producers and making sure that they came from within a 40-mile radius of the city. In order to draw in a wider variety of stallholders, however, they decided to be less rigid about whether or not produce was organic.

The rewards

The Bath Farmers' Market continues to thrive today, and it has acted as an important venue for local projects such as the Broadlands Community Orchard (described on page 95). Transition City Bath is another local group which has a stall at the market-place once a month to help maintain awareness of its presence in the community. In the early months of 2009 Keith noticed a considerable rise in the footfall at the market (which he estimates to be as much as 40 per cent higher than in 2008), and he puts this down to the fact that consumers are tired of a global food system that "pulls the wool over their eyes" and that they are now actively looking for fresher, healthier food direct from the local people who produce it. The fact that this is happening at the time of an economic downturn indicates that, at least for the shoppers in Bath, global financial insecurity doesn't have to imply local food insecurity.

Project name: Wolverton Farmers' Market

Location: Wolverton, near Milton Keynes

Aim: To re-establish a farmers' market to provide residents with fresh, local produce and to promote local food issues in general.

Started: 2004

How many people involved: Six volunteers, one paid market manager, twelve stallholders and an average of 500 customers on market day.

On the web: www.foodtrain.org.uk

The idea

One farmers' market to have sprung up in the wake of Bath's success was that in Wolverton on the outskirts of Milton Keynes. Wolverton is itself a small town

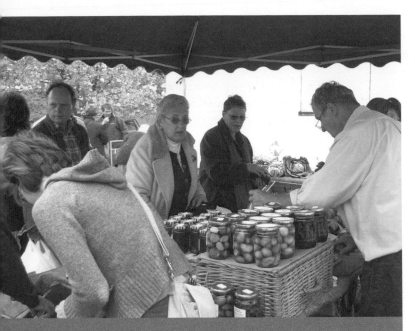

A stall at the Wolverton Farmers' Market. Photograph: Food Train

The action

A team of seven residents set about organising the events – one planned for harvest time and the other at Christmas. They scoured other nearby markets for potential stallholders, chatting to producers and giving them the chance to try out the two pilots before committing to the Wolverton market on a more permanent basis. All in all, they managed to pull in twenty-five stallholders.

Both pilot markets were very successful and popular with consumers and producers alike, so the team decided to schedule bimonthly markets for the following year. When working to source local producers for the stalls, Alissa and others realised that setting a limit of a 30-mile radius would be too difficult in their area, and that it would exclude a free-range butcher they were keen to have on board. So they chose to set the limit at 50 miles instead. Like the founders of the Bath Farmers' Market, they are keen to promote organic, pesticide-free produce but not exclusively, and they do include non-organic foods too. The Wolverton team has also chosen to increase market variety and extend its definition of ethical produce beyond the local by including a stall that's run by a Fairtrade shop in Milton Keynes.

The way it works

In 2006, the market's founders set up the organisation Food Train as a limited company and a social enterprise, with the aim of running the Wolverton market and exploring ways of improving local food availability in the area. Since receiving the initial start-up funding for the farmers' market, the project as a whole has been run entirely on the small budget drawn from stall rentals. This pays for the market manager's wages, while any surplus profit is put back into Food Train and used to cover the cost of gazebos, signage

with a population of about 9,000, but it is slowly being subsumed by its neighbouring city. It was a thriving market town up until the 1980s, when a large Tesco store moved in and the market soon moved out.

Some years later, in 2003, the Countryside Agency (a statutory body now known as Natural England) funded a project to explore how the people of Wolverton could create sustainable community enterprises in their town. As part of the project, local people were asked to participate in a visioning process to help generate ideas. Local resident Alissa Pemberton, inspired by a bustling farmers' market she had visited on a trip to Canada, suggested that they work to bring back a local food market in Wolverton. The idea received the support it needed from other residents, and the Agency agreed to fund two pilot markets to get the project off the ground.

and other market materials. All other work is done by Alissa and other volunteers. They now have twelve core producers (including the local WI group), selling honey, eggs, cakes, breads, red meat and organic fruit and vegetables, and between them have a turnover of approximately £1,500 per market.

The challenges

Since its initial burst of success the market has experienced a drop in stall numbers and consumers. There are a few possible reasons for this fall in trade, including the ever-dominant presence of the Tesco supermarket and the fact that Wolverton Farmers' Market receives little passing custom but is mainly attended by committed local people. But the Food Train team is determined to keep the market on its toes, and is constantly working to get the right mix of stalls and to promote the market as much as possible in the local community.

Beyond the Wolverton Farmers' Market

Food Train's experience in running the market, sourcing producers and piecing together an overall picture of local food production in the area has led its members to look at ways of filling the local food gaps that the market has exposed. In contrast to the situation in Bath, they have found it hard to find a good variety of producers because much of the food production in the Milton Keynes area serves the commodity market instead of feeding the people in the surrounding communities. So, with much inspiration and help from the London-based food project Growing Communities (described in Chapter 14), Food Train and its partner the Milton Keynes Christian Foundation are now working on developing a project called the Urb Farm on a 4-acre site in Wolverton. There, food is being grown just feet away from where it will be consumed. Organic and no-dig methods are being used, and there is a strong emphasis on community engagement from local schools, gardening groups and willing volunteers from the public. Once the Urb Farm is harvesting at full swing, the market can act as one of the outlets for its produce, which will also be sold through a farm shop and in a cafe on the farm site.

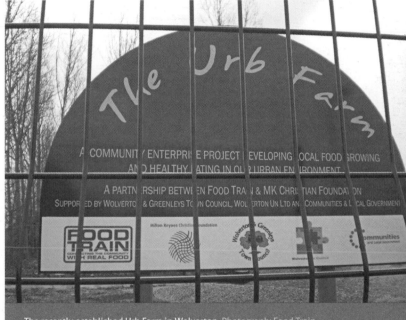

The recently established Urb Farm in Wolverton. Photograph: Food Train

The development of local food work in Wolverton is yet another example of how one local food project can generate enough interest and attention to give rise to other related elements of a growing local food network. Because Food Train was created to support the wider principles of local food production, the farmers' market project was never intended to be a destination in itself, but a stepping-stone towards greater food resilience in the area. Food Train's work pre-dated the emergence of Transition Town Wolverton (which was established in May 2008), but their shared aims of building and promoting food security mean that they both benefit from a joining of forces.

Project name: Redland Farmers' Market

Location: Redland, Bristol

Aim: To raise awareness about local food issues, make local produce easily available for local people, and to create a regular community event that has sustainability at its core.

Started: 2006

How many people involved: One market manager, up to seven volunteers, eighteen to twenty stallholders and hundreds of customers on market day.

On the web: www.sustainableredland.org.uk

The idea

Back in the south-west of England, another farmers' market has been helping to nurture a rise in food-security awareness while satisfying the growing appetite for local produce that accompanies it. The Sustainable Redland group was formed when local resident Hamish Wills took it upon himself to write and deliver a letter to other Redland homes, inviting others to join him in creating a positive-focused, proactive environmental initiative in their community. After an initial meeting, Sustainable Redland sprang into being in 2005, signing up as a Transition initiative in 2007. One of its first projects was to establish a farmers' market, something that resident Jonny Wood had wanted to initiate for some time, and for which he found new impetus through the encouragement of other Sustainable Redland members.

Organising a farmers' market was a new challenge for the Sustainable Redland team, whose members' enthusiasm outweighed their experience, so they looked outside the group for some market-savvy assistance. Jonny got in touch with Jim Wilkie, the manager of the nearby and recently established Fishponds Market, for advice. Jim was keen to help and it was agreed that he would take on the management role for the Redland Farmers' Market as well. His experience in matters such as booking the site, arranging the necessary permissions and licences, and knowing how to pull in a good selection of stallholders from his existing contacts has proven extremely valuable.

The action

The first market didn't generate as many producers or customers as the team had hoped, but by the second one the numbers of both had doubled. The market now has, on average, twenty stalls – 80 per cent of which have a regular presence. But, according to Jonny, there is something new there each time, and, as long as there is always a balanced variety of produce, space can be made for new producers to come on board. At the time of writing the market is run every two weeks, though it may yet grow and become more frequent.

Because they didn't go for any funding, Jonny and company covered the initial start-up costs themselves – but these weren't huge. The market is situated on a church forecourt and the landlords agreed that rent could be paid retrospectively after six months. So after the first two markets (when traders were enticed in with the offer of free stall space), the stall rental was set at a price that would cover the rent, Jim's wages, insurance and electricity bills. Beyond that, the costs of advertising the project through posters, and the time taken to make all the necessary arrangements and phone calls, were taken by the Sustainable Redlanders. Like the Wolverton Farmers' Market described on page 117, Redland now operates as a social enterprise and no profit is made that doesn't go back into the project.

In order to carry out its commitment to local food, the Redland Farmers' Market has traders sourced only from within a 50-mile radius, and the stallholder must also be the producer. It is Jim's role to ensure that no traders are acting as middlemen for other producers, and that all food labelled as 'organic' is certified. Jim also has a team of volunteer assistants (from Sustainable Redland and the wider local community) who help to set up and tidy up the site, and to keep the traders happy and the kettle regularly boiling.

In order to help spread the availability of local produce, the team has tried to build good relationships with the local shopkeepers. Some of the nearby shops now source products from the traders at the market, and in return the market helps to draw more people and passing custom to the area. Because it has become a focal point of community life, the market also provides Sustainable Redland with an opportunity for promoting its work, events, and its vision of community resilience.

The rewards

Looking back on the process from the original idea to the first few months of trading, Jonny sees it as having been hugely satisfying – and also relatively easy. He has been fortunate to have found a good site, a supportive market manager and a receptive audience, but Sustainable Redland's success is also evidence that setting up a farmers' market can be an effective way of tapping into, gathering together and feeding a community's support for local food.

Tips on setting up a farmers' market

As suggested by Peter Andrews (Bath), Alissa Pemberton (Food Train), Jonny Wood (Sustainable Redland) and Bethan Stagg (community scientist, Totnes).

1. Start by doing the necessary research. It may well be that your community already has good access to local food and that a market is not the most suitable vehicle for promoting local produce. Also find out whether potential local producers are keen on the idea of a new market. Some may feel that they attend enough market days as it is, and others may prefer not to pack up and transport their produce if there is no guarantee that they will make a decent enough profit – in which case a CSA-type structure (see Chapter 8) might suit them much better.

2. Finding someone with a good deal of experience in running markets is a great help and cuts down on the time needed to research and make contacts.

3. Try to avoid holding the first market in winter (especially in the post-Christmas slump), midsummer, or at other quieter times.

4. Wander around other farmers' markets in the area to get an idea of what stalls work well, what would make your market unique, and to make sure you don't closely replicate what others do, or clash with events (e.g. tastings, themed festivals) they might be holding.

5. If possible, try to make sure the market's site is visible and easily accessible, with nearby toilet, parking, washing and electrical facilities, and perhaps that it is even weather-proof. The site can also benefit from being close to other food

shops, partly because of mutual support but also because the shops and stalls can combine to be a good alternative to the supermarket.

6. Find out whether planning permission is required for your chosen site. It will be necessary for some sites and not for others.

7. If local shop traders are apprehensive about the market's presence, it might be a good idea to suggest having a stall at the market promoting some of the local shops. Making the effort to get these traders on board may well be worthwhile from the market's point of view, so do persist.

8. Choosing what day of the week the market is to run on can greatly affect customer numbers. A 'good market day' will vary across different communities, depending upon other local, weekly and/or seasonal happenings (such as other markets or festivals). Liaising with the council can help to minimise clashes.

9. Keep the market's hours short and sweet. If the market runs for too long it can mean refrigeration or chill boxes are necessary for some products, which can become complicated.

10. Make sure the needs of stallholders and customers are heard: this will contribute to a stronger sense of engagement with and commitment to the market. There are many ways of doing this, from conducting questionnaires to simple chatting and making cups of coffee – or, if appropriate, forming an elected management committee from among the stallholders to oversee the project.

11. The market can be used as a showcase for local entertainers, and to promote other local sustainability projects – both of which can help to establish the market as a hub for community life.

Having a regular table or noticeboard for fund-raising and advertising upcoming events can be helpful.

12. Keep up regular checks on the producers' organic and hygiene certificates to ensure the market's reputation remains intact.

13. Have a team of volunteer helpers: this gives local residents the opportunity to be part of the market, while also helping to keep costs down.

14. Try to link up with other organisations that may be interested in supporting a local farmers' market, such as social services, chambers of commerce, environmental organisations and producers groups, e.g. FARMA, the National Farmers' Union (NFU) and regional organisations such as Taste of the West.

15. Use your market as a catalyst for greater local food action in the community. A farmers' market can be a useful gauge of a community's willingness to buy local, and can also be an outlet for other local food projects that it can help to inspire and provide custom for (such as a small-scale commercial herb garden or a jam-making cooperative that could sell its produce at the market).

Resources

See page 195 for Farmers' markets and page 197 for Funding, grants and loans.

Chapter 10

FOOD COOPERATIVES

The themes of shared ownership and decision-making that cut across many of the initiatives featured in this book are most clearly demonstrated by food cooperative projects, which have a concern with organisational structure at their core. These projects emphasise the importance not only of 'what' we eat but also 'how' we organise ourselves around access to it.

In its simplest form, a cooperative is a group of people who draw together, in equal capacity, with a common purpose – whether it is to sell, buy or provide a service.[1]

At the heart of the cooperative approach is an ethic of respect for fellow members, be they workers (as in a textile company owned by its employees), customers (such as a supermarket owned by consumers) or both. In this model, responsibility, ownership and power are shared among members for their mutual benefit, helping to nurture a strong sense of commitment to the enterprise and the principles it upholds. The way cooperatives go about achieving this varies a lot, depending on the context. Smaller cooperatives with simpler aims (such as a chicken co-op owned and run collectively by five families) do of course have far less need for formality and have more direct access to decision-making procedures than, say, a national bank that has millions of customers. Some have consensus-based, 'flat structures' while others are more hierarchical but democratic (where, for example, a management committee is elected by other members). But

they are all set up to serve people rather than stock-exchange listings, shareholder profits and the odd swollen pension – they are about striving for true worker and/or customer satisfaction.

This emphasis on 'people care' often supports a culture in which a wider sense of 'care' can grow, so that many cooperatives also choose to operate within the boundaries of human rights and environmental sustainability – using products, energy and other resources from as 'clean' and 'cruelty-free' sources as possible, and encouraging their customers to do the same. For the ethics of care to be thoroughly and genuinely upheld, it simply makes sense that they are reflected in the structures that promote them – then they are visible, tangible actions instead of just promising words.

Food co-ops in the UK enjoyed a flurry of activity in the 1960s and 1970s, but they then hit a supermarket-driven lull in popularity that has only recently been revived. Their current resurgence has much to do with rising food prices, and many of them are located in deprived areas of the country. But the growing number of these groups is also a result of the linked threats of community breakdown and food insecurity, something that co-op members can help ward off by pooling their energies to source local, organic food between them. At the same time, more co-ops are choosing to deal directly with producers for some or all of their procurement needs, instead of sourcing all of their food from centralised wholesalers.

Broadly, food cooperatives could be said to include any food project that is organised 'cooperatively' (including some Community Supported Agriculture schemes, community gardens and farmers' markets). But for the purpose of this book we focus on those that source and distribute local and/or organic food (as opposed to growing or processing it). By drawing together the buying power and community interest of their consumer-members, these food co-ops are able to keep food prices down while also supporting more sustainable forms of food production. In so doing, they are reclaiming food supply chains, strengthening cooperative links within a community, forming direct relationships with producers while providing them with a reliable market, and bypassing the costly overheads of the centralised 'middlemen'. Beyond these similarities, they vary in size (from small buying groups that source only what their members order to bigger initiatives that operate markets and shops), in member choice (from being able to pick individual items of a sale or order to choosing between standard selections of fruit and vegetables), how they are organised (from informal, collection-point arrangements between friends to legally registered, home-delivery businesses) and how frequently they operate (anything from daily to annually).

While all the projects described in the following pages have an active awareness of the relationship between food and community resilience, they go about facilitating that link in different ways. Some prioritise 'organic' over 'local', and vice versa. But the more food cooperatives within this movement expand their efforts into sourcing both local and organic food, the more they will encourage a market for such produce, with the infrastructure and jobs needed to support it. At the same time, the way they are organised and run has important implications for how we

can share communication, work, decision-making and of course food in the transition to a community-engaged food culture.

Food cooperative stories

Project name: Food For All
Location: Hartcliffe, Bristol
Aim: To provide local residents with affordable, local, largely organic food.
Started: 1991
How many people involved: Over 200 household members
On the web: www.foodforallbristol.org.uk

The idea

The Food For All cooperative, which operates in Bristol's Hartcliffe area, is an example of a well-established co-op committed to supplying affordable food to local residents, and one that has recently transformed its procurement policy to favour local and organic produce. Back in 1990, Hartcliffe was the subject of a survey conducted by local health authorities, who concluded that the area was seriously deprived; that, among other issues, unemployment was worryingly high and shop closures were making it very hard for residents to access affordable, nutritious food. These observations made by objective onlookers struck a community chord and inspired change from within, triggering the formation of the Hartcliffe Health and Environment Action Group (HHEAG), set up and run by local residents. One of HHEAG's earliest projects was to come up with a way of getting affordable, decent food to Hartcliffe residents

Food co-ops
Kath Dalmeny

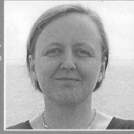

Photograph: Sustain

Increasingly, people are setting up food co-ops so they can get good food at an affordable price, by benefiting from economies of scale in purchasing and transporting food. Buying food cooperatively could play a key role in helping to reduce fuel use and oil dependence in the food system, so co-ops are a very useful tool for Transition Towns. Food co-ops can also be a good way for communities to make direct relationships with farmers, ensuring a reliable supply of fresh seasonal food and a reliable income for the people who grow it.

Since food is something that we all need, every day, running a food co-op can provide great opportunities for people to meet each other, learn new skills and make a positive contribution to their community.

Our new food co-ops webpage, www.sustainweb.org/foodcoops (funded by the Big Lottery via the Making Local Food Work programme, and created by the food and farming charity Sustain), can help you find out if there's already a food co-op to join in your area. Or, if not, it will give you all the information you need to set up your own. You can also sign up to a newsletter to receive information and news about relevant events, publications and funding opportunities.

Kath Dalmeny is a food campaigner and the policy director for Sustain, a London-based alliance of public-interest organisations working for greater sustainability in food and farming (see www.sustainweb.org, and its new webpage www.sustainweb.org/foodcoops for a co-op directory and to download the Food Co-op toolkit).

– and the co-op buying model provided the simplest and most cost-effective solution.

The action

The co-op was set up under the name Food For All, and, as the name suggests, its primary goal is to make food accessible to everyone in the community, whatever their income. Over the years it has steadily grown to become a successful co-op serving over 200 households through its shop and outreach stalls held in various community venues. Membership is open only to residents of the BS13 area, who pay £2 a year entitling them to a 10 per cent discount on all co-op products. Non-residents and non-co-op members are, however, welcome to buy produce in the shop but don't receive the same discount. Once someone becomes a member, he or she is encouraged (but not forced!) to undertake voluntary duties at the co-op, from pricing products to advertising the project locally, as well as being given the necessary training. There are two paid workers managing the shop and the stalls respectively, but all other work is carried out by volunteers. The co-op is a non-profit-making social enterprise and, while it has relied on funding for specific projects (such as to help set up the shop), it is, on the whole, self-sufficient. Decision-making is in the hands of the management committee (which is comprised of seven people), elected at each AGM by fellow members.

Once a working mechanism was in place for getting affordable food to local residents, the Food For All team began looking at ways of reducing the environmental impact of the business by cutting its dependency on fossil-fuelled food miles and encouraging residents to support local food producers. It has since built up a group of suppliers that reflect its commitment to local, organic agriculture, including HHEAG's own Greens Community Garden, Leigh Court Farm and the Alvis Brothers' meat and dairy farm. Through HHEAG's other work, Food For All is linked with a network of local-food-focused initiatives, such as their educational Pot to Plate food programme, and the Sow and Grow community gardening courses.

Sue Walker, who has worked with HHEAG and on the Food For All project for fifteen years, observes that their work is hugely rewarding but that their spare time is limited. Because of this, links with the burgeoning Transition City Bristol groups are yet to be established. But their work is 'Transition' by another name, as they help their community to reconnect with the importance of nutritious, safe food grown near to home. This co-op is an example of a node of local food activity that Transition and other community food groups can learn and draw inspiration from. Because it operates in such a deprived inner-city area, its success

is yet more evidence[1] of the fact that a tightening of the purse strings does not have to imply a rejection of food ethics – the two are compatible and, in the name of post-oil sustainability, entirely necessary. We *can* have our affordable, local, organic cake and eat it too.

Project name: The Fruit and Veg Together Co-op

Location: Milton, Westcliff, Essex

Aim: To provide local residents with weekly, fresh, organic produce distributed at a collection point.

Started: March 2008

How many people involved: One to two volunteers, up to fifty households.

Transition initiative website: www.westclifftransition. wordpress.com

The idea

At the other end of the food co-op scale in terms of size, formality and age is the Fruit and Veg Together Co-op, running in the deprived Milton area of Westcliff, Essex – also home to the active Transition Town Westcliff group. This initiative offers a helpful comparison with Food For All's work, described from page 124, because it gives a snapshot idea of how such a project might look in its early days. As is often the case, the Fruit and Veg Together Co-op was the brainchild of motivated individuals, determined to extend their commitment to local food to other members of their community.

Louise Harris had previous experience of being in a food cooperative when she moved to Westcliff in 2008, and she began wondering about how to set one up in her new community. She decided to get in touch with local charity the Milton Community Partnership, established in the late 1990s to encourage self-

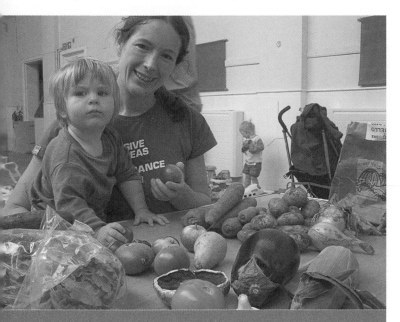

At the Fruit and Veg Together collection in Transition Town Westcliff.
Photograph: Transition Town Westcliff

Eleanor the chance to get feedback from participants, to determine how much volunteer help was needed to help run the project, and to plan how to take things further. Following on from the pilot, the co-op team decided to hold a member recruitment event where free samples of fruit and vegetables from a few different suppliers were given out, and responses to them were compared.

Some months on, the project now has fifty members who buy their fruit and vegetables through the co-op – some weekly and others less frequently. There is a choice of four different bags that members pay for and order a week in advance. Unlike the Food For All Co-op (see page 124), there is no membership fee, since it is a much smaller enterprise, and customers simply pay for their ordered produce. Eleanor now runs the project herself and, with occasional help from other volunteers, she bags the fruit and vegetables up each week before they are collected by co-op customers – either from a local after-school club or from Eleanor's home.

determination and reconnection within the community. There she found support for her idea in the shape of Eleanor King, a member of Transition Town Westcliff. Between them, Louise and Eleanor conducted a survey of Milton residents to assess the need for increased access to local, organic food in the area. The response was overwhelmingly positive and, with evidence of local support for her plans, Louise and Eleanor went about organising a trial run of the food co-op model.

The action

Twelve willing participants were recruited for the trial, each of whom agreed to pay £3 a week for a bag of fruit and £3 for a bag of vegetables sourced from a local, organic wholesaler. This pilot run gave Louise and

The challenges

After the produce-sampling session, the River Nene organic box scheme in East Anglia was chosen as the co-op's suppliers. This choice does stretch the definition of 'local produce' because their fruit and vegetables are either grown on a farm over 100 miles away in Peterborough, or imported (though not air-freighted) in Britain's hungrier seasons. But this decision was made in the face of a number of tricky questions that are familiar to many community food projects, such as: Where does the 'local' boundary lie? Is 'local' to be prioritised over and above considerations of organics, quality, choice and price? And is it acceptable to settle for distantly sourced produce as luxury items or as a temporary measure before local food networks are fully established?

In short, the co-op's choice to buy food in over-county lines highlights the difficulties that community projects can be confronted with when trying to balance customer satisfaction with the principles of sustainable food production and procurement. It also reflects the reality that we are in the midst of a shift from a global to a local food system, and this is a time when a variety of approaches to food sourcing are being tried and tested before the ethics of planetary and human health can converge. Eleanor and other co-op members chose River Nene because it can supply smaller amounts of specific products when orders are low, provides good-quality, organic produce, accepts Healthy Start vouchers, reuses its bags and offers free delivery. This is certainly a move in the right direction (Milton is after all much closer to Peterborough than it is to Jujuy, Argentina) and one that opens up a space for local residents to explore the meaning of 'good food', where it comes from and how it's grown. But, as the co-op is fully aware, it does have some way to go before 'food miles' are replaced by 'food metres', and before Milton residents can be certain that the effects of peak oil will not leave them hungry. Part of Eleanor's and others' future plans therefore include running workshops and giving out seedlings and seeds to encourage residents to grow their own, and they also have visions of establishing an organic farm in their area.

The rewards

An unexpected, positive outcome of the co-op's work is the community dimension of collectively buying and picking up food. Eleanor has noticed many food-related conversations developing at the collection point, and a growing awareness around matters of food production, healthy eating and home cooking. The co-op's presence at the after-school club has encouraged members to spend more time there talking to others, so that a thriving hub of food-focused residents is being nurtured. Eleanor has also used the co-op's foothold in the community as a way of promoting related events and groups (including Transition Town Westcliff) by putting leaflets in with the fruit and vegetable bags.

Project name: Wellington Food Cooperative

Location: Wellington, Somerset

Aim: To provide very locally produced, fresh food in season from small suppliers in and around Wellington, to support local suppliers to expand their production, and to encourage Wellington people to eat local, seasonal produce.

Started: June 2007

How many people involved: Two organisers, approximately ninety members and six producers.

The idea

Unlike the group in Westcliff described above, the following food co-op is fortunate enough to have a good choice of local food producers in its area, and the direct support of local agriculture is at the heart of its principles. Wellington Food Cooperative was started up by Taunton Borough Council to encourage young mothers to eat more healthily. But after three months funding was withdrawn from the project and it was left to its own devices. Holly Regan-Jones, who has more recently helped to initiate the Transition Town Wellington initiative, became involved with the co-op as a food access worker, and when the funding dried up she decided to continue running the project herself.

The action

Holly had no background experience in food supply, but was drawn to the co-op's work because of her own interest in local food and her desire to be part of building food resilience in her area. When she took on the running of the co-op the local vegetable and meat producers were already on board, but she has since added other producers to the list of suppliers, including a fishmonger, an apple-juice producer and a fruit farm – all of whom (except the fishmonger, who is permitted extra mileage because of the town's distance from the coast) operate within 20 miles of the town. They are all organic, but none of them is certified. Holly now receives help in running the co-op from local vegetable grower Ray Weymouth, who also sells his produce through the scheme.

The co-op has two drop-off times in different venues in Wellington – one during the day at a children's centre and the other in the evening at a local youth centre. Members don't pay a joining fee but they pay weekly for their produce, choosing between three sizes of fruit and vegetable selections, costing £6, £8 and £10, each week. They can also order apple juice and a range of fish and meat products when these are available. They collect their weekly produce (which they find in a bucket with their membership number on the front) and pay and order for the following week based on what the producers have in season. The co-op makes a little profit from the apple juice it sells, which is put back into the project, but all other produce is sold for no profit and Holly and Ray give their time voluntarily.

One important lesson that Holly and Ray have learned through running the Wellington Food Co-op is that the location of the collection point venue can greatly affect public awareness of a co-op's work and how successfully it recruits members. The children's centre collection point is more popular and developed a larger membership base much more quickly than the evening scheme. Holly attributes this to the fact that the former has much passing custom and is in a prominent position in town. The timing of the collection point is also a factor, and the slot at the children's centre receives more attention because it is held during busier, daylight hours.

Beyond the members who were part of the co-op's original set-up, Holly has recruited new customers through the co-op's contacts with local health visitors, and through putting up permanent posters, placing articles in the local paper and holding a stall at the Food Fair in the summer. The co-op's vegetable grower also advertises the project through leaflets on his monthly stall at the local farmers' market. As part of the drive to draw in new members, Holly has done a cost comparison between the co-op's produce and similar items found at the nearby Tesco and Sainsbury's supermarkets. She found the co-op's prices to be considerably lower, which has comforted existing members and encouraged more to sign up. In fact, Holly has found, through speaking with members, that many of them now actively avoid shopping at supermarkets since they've been part of the co-op, and that they have changed their attitudes to food, health and their connection with local agriculture.

The rewards

Holly finds the running of the co-op fun and satisfying, and has already seen its work have a positive effect on local producers. The co-op's vegetable grower, for example, has been able to increase his production and purchase a new field as a result of the guaranteed weekly custom he receives through the project. Ray and Holly are keen to help spread the co-op word and have already assisted two new, nearby co-ops in setting up their books. They also see their food project as a potential outlet for raising Transition awareness in the town and as having an important role in strengthening local food supply.

Some closing thoughts on food cooperatives

Beyond the food co-op approaches described here there is the added option of turning such a project into a web-based enterprise – something that can still be done without entirely replacing social interaction with screens and keyboard clicks. One project that is a thriving example of this approach is found in Oklahoma in the US. There, Robert Waldrop has built up a cooperative (almost entirely self-financed by food sales) that now takes online sales of 60-70,000 dollars each month, from its 2,000-plus members (see www. oklahomafood.coop and www.localfoodcoop.org).

However food co-ops are run and whatever scale they work on, their ability to help pool the resources of time, money, social connections, transport and work is what makes them particularly appropriate to the energy descent we are embarking on. This kind of sharing within the community will be a necessary and potentially positive feature of life in a fossil-fuel-lean society, for which many local food co-ops are already well equipped.

Tips on setting up a food cooperative

As suggested by Sue Walker (Food For All), Eleanor King (Fruit and Veg Together Co-op), and Holly Regan-Jones (Wellington Food Cooperative).

1. Building a community-run project such as a food co-op is about forging connections and strengthening relationships within a community – which can take a great deal of time. So patience is required in preparing the ground (for example, through community open-space events or workshops) and nurturing further growth of the project (until the membership limit is reached and workers can then consider helping other co-ops to set up too!).

2. Internet research is one way of identifying local producers to work with, and some countries and regions are lucky enough to have websites listing local food businesses in their area. But it is also worth exploring other ways of finding them, as some smaller businesses may well not be listed on the web. Check out local food directories and ads in local papers, and chat to other residents, independent shopkeepers and stallholders at nearby farmers' markets.

3. You can also be creative about ways of recruiting customer-members – by, for example, holding food events where people can come and meet the co-op farmers and sample their produce, having a recruitment stall at a farmers' market or providing the food for another public event (such as a Transition Town talk or film screening). Places and groups to advertise through include health-food shops, doctors' surgeries, churches, restaurants, alternative health clinics, crèches, and any Transition-, peak-oil- or climate-change-related organisations.

4. Experience in setting up a co-op is helpful, but certainly not a prerequisite for running a successful food co-op initiative. Check out other nearby co-ops for advice, tips and maybe even ongoing support. And don't underestimate the willingness of members to chip in with ideas, labour, materials

and venues – it is their co-op and they have a vested interest in seeing it thrive.

5. Regularly consult members on their opinions of the co-op's work so that they can have input into, and ownership over, the project. Be flexible enough to be able to respond to members' desire for change, which may include anything from switching to more local producers, asking co-op farmers to certify their land, finding ways of operating a packaging-free business or extending the range of products.

6. If you choose to operate a collection scheme, be sure to research possible venues and time slots carefully by visiting the area at the times in question to see how much passing pedestrian traffic there is. You can also check out whether times coincide with any other weekly happenings in the same venue or nearby (such as mother-and-baby classes, etc.), and canvas potential or existing members to find out what time and location suit them best.

7. Co-ops can be a useful mechanism for spreading information about related local projects, such as Transition initiatives, gardening workshops, etc., and thereby helping to link local food work in the area. Because local food co-ops can be an effective entry point into a wider appreciation of food security issues, you can help to nurture this awareness among members by providing informa-tion on home growing, sharing listings of related local workshops and courses, and directing them towards other ways of accessing organic local food.

Resources

See page 197 for Food co-ops and Funding, grants and loans, and page 203 for Local food – general.

Chapter 11

LOCAL FOOD GUIDES AND DIRECTORIES

As described in Chapter 1, the local food sector is currently enjoying a welcome revival in the UK and abroad. But there is still much that can be done to improve access to local produce, encourage more consumers to choose it, and ensure that this revival keeps on rolling. One popular way for community groups to support a growing preference for local foods is by compiling a guide or directory that will point consumers in the direction of the producers, shops, restaurants, cafes and gardens that can provide them with the local, healthy, affordable and safe food they need. Having such a guide helps to demystify the world of local food buying for the shopper, while giving local businesses the opportunity to promote their wares in the immediate community.

One of the first local food directories to be compiled in the UK was the *Forest Food Directory*, with listings of local food producers and retailers in the Forest of Dean, Gloucestershire. Written by Matt Dunwell and Kate de Selincourt, this directory soon grabbed the attention of other local food supporters around the country and inspired many others to work on similar projects (including some of the Transition folk in Totnes, as described later). You can read more about Matt's perspective on the project below.

In putting together a directory of local food, you will inevitably come up against some of the murky definitions and ethical boundaries that this particular food sector throws up (as discussed on pages 21-22). How do we define local and regional food? How do we classify a business as being a local food business? And do supermarkets selling local produce deserve to be included in local food listings? It is up to community groups grappling with these issues to come up with their own answers to these and other local food questions. But it is important that whatever definitions or decisions you arrive at are explained and made clear to your readers. Define what you mean by local, organic, regional, etc., and why you are listing some businesses while omitting others. That way, the baton is handed back to consumers, who can then make their own shopping choices based on the transparent information you provide them with.

The Forest Food Directory

Matt Dunwell

Photograph: Matt Dunwell

Back in early 1997 it was quite hard to source local food unless you knew the farmer or spotted a roadside sign. There were no farmers' markets until later that year and local food was still a small niche.

The Forest of Dean in Gloucestershire had a good range of local growers and, at a Local Agenda 21 meeting, Kate de Selincourt and myself proposed that we map farmers and growers who were providing for the local market, and create a Local Food Directory.

We asked the farms we wanted to list in the directory whether they would accept farm visits at least once a year. Most were more than happy to, and this tended to make sure the first edition was populated with the small, family-oriented farms. We then listed the products and opening times of each.

It is hard to police a food directory – we didn't have the money or inclination to become a licensing body. Instead Kate and I wrote short articles for the directory in the hope that people would ask farmers and growers about topics such as the local economy and why it is good to shop locally, food miles, packaging and animal welfare. We also included a piece on the role small farmers have played over the centuries in providing and preserving genetic diversity. We hoped this would help consumers ask pertinent questions and keep the growers on their toes.

It is difficult to assess the impact of the directory, as it coincided with an expansion of the local food sector across the board. There were growers who said it made a large difference to their turnover, and those who were indifferent. Personally, I think it helped to identify the Forest of Dean as a local food destination, and to forge links with the District Council, who helped with the printing and were supportive of our work. We now have the Forest Food Showcase event every year, which goes from strength to strength. The lesson for me is that it is relatively easy to get farmers and growers together and put them in a directory, but getting them to work together is the Holy Grail, as they have so little time spare for group marketing activity. A food producers group did emerge here in the early 2000s, but it struggled to get going and has now fallen apart. I always feel that the French tendency to encourage grower cooperation has served them well and so I hope to one day see more of that happening over here.

Matt Dunwell is a permaculture designer, publisher and teacher. He runs courses from Ragmans Farm in the Forest of Dean, Gloucestershire (see www.ragmans.co.uk).

Local food guide and directory stories

Project name: A Celebration of Local Food – The Totnes guide to local food, shopping and eating out

Location: Totnes, Devon

Aim: To promote businesses, producers and retailers of local food, and to make it easier for consumers to support their local economy by sourcing food locally.

Started: September 2006

How many people involved: Six volunteers

On the web: www.totnes.transitionnetwork.org/localfooddirectory/home

The idea

Noni Mackenzie has been an active supporter of local food for many years, having run her own local food shop until 2000. Once the shop closed, she was keen to do something else to support her small-scale producer contacts and friends in the area, all of whom were struggling to keep their heads above water.

Inspired by the success of the Forest of Dean local food directory (see page 133), Noni began entertaining the idea of drawing together a local food guide for Totnes, to promote local produce and show consumers where it could be found. At about the same time, Transition Town Totnes (TTT) was unleashed on the community, and Noni found the impetus she needed for her idea through attending talks, watching the film *The Power of Community* and participating in Open Space events. It was at the Energy Open Space event that she decided to share her food-guide plans, and she left out lists for interested people (producers and business owners, as well as for willing volunteers) to

fill in their contact details. Lists were also put out at the organic veg stall in the weekly market, and it was not long before Noni found some enthusiastic collaborators and the local food-guide group was formed.

The cover of the Totnes guide to local food, shopping and eating out. Photograph: Transition Town Totnes

The action

Noni and the rest of the group met and chatted through their plans for the project, and it was decided to run a pilot in the directory's first year, following this up with a public evaluation before pushing forward with an official version. They shared the tasks of chatting with businesses up and down the high street and around the town, quizzing them on their local, organic food credentials, their contact information and their opening times.

There were of course a number of grey areas that had to be navigated when deciding what businesses to include in the guide. The team chose, for instance, not to include the town's large supermarket in the listings for the reason that most of its revenue is siphoned away from the local economy. It also decided to restrict its research to Totnes proper, which excluded a large-scale local organic farm a few miles away but ensured a clear boundary for the work. Much heated debate was involved before arriving at these decisions, but mutual agreement was eventually reached.

Although the group put a firm boundary in place by deciding to keep the supermarket out, it tried to encourage consumer choice regarding all the other local businesses included in the guide. This was done by placing symbols alongside listed businesses to indicate whether they sold food sourced from within 5 miles of Totnes, within South Devon, and/or from the south-west of England; whether food sold was organic, biodynamic or labelled by the Wholesome Food Association (which provides an affordable, trust-based form of organic accreditation); and whether the business accepted TTT's local currency, the Totnes Pound. The group also included a map of Totnes (on to which businesses were plotted), local recipes written up by local people, a number of articles on local food and specially commissioned drawings by local artist Jane Warring.

The whole thrust of the publication is clearly in favour of local food (as evidenced by its title *A Celebration of Local Food*), but by including all the town's food-related businesses (supermarket aside) it encourages informed decision-making while recognising that the local food market operates within the complex world of consumer choice – and that local produce makes up only one part of the local economy the group also wanted to support. Another decision made by the group to support consumer choice was in the naming of the project. The publication was called a 'guide' rather than a 'directory' to emphasise to readers that they were being guided, rather than directed in the way its creators thought they should go.

Keeping consumer perspective and freedom of choice in mind, the team decided not to take on any advertising to fund the project. Its members felt that this would have unfairly prioritised the more prosperous businesses in the town, instead of giving each one equal space. So they chose to try to fund the printing and design costs of the pilot run (£2,000 and £500 respectively) by applying for a grant from the National Lottery's Awards for All scheme. When the application for the grant was delayed, a generous local benefactor had to step in at the last minute to ensure that the project would go ahead. This meant that the group was able to print up 3,000 copies ready for the launch event. When they did eventually receive the grant, they were able to put the benefactor's money towards their next, official publication.

The guide and the Totnes Pound (see page 170 for more about food and local currencies) were launched by the town mayor in the Totnes market square, in a celebration of all things local.

After the launch, copies were made available for free in local shops and at the market, the Tourist Information Centre and various TTT events, and they were eagerly snapped up. Just one year later, the team produced its official and updated version of the guide, which made space for more information on local producers as well as including information on seasonal produce and how to get involved in local food work. This time, however, the decision was made to charge for the publication to give it greater value, and the team has since managed to raise more than £500 from sales, which will be put towards local food initiatives. Beyond its importance for the community of Totnes, the official guide has also been spread widely among other Transition initiatives keen to work on similar projects of their own.

Project name: The Glastonbury Local Food Directory

Location: Glastonbury, Somerset

Aim: To publish a directory of local producers and retailers of local food.

Started: September 2007

How many people involved: Four to five

Transition initiative website: www.transitiontowns. org/glastonbury

The idea

The food group of Transition Town Glastonbury, inspired by above project in Totnes, decided to go about producing its own local food directory in September 2007. Unlike the Totnes group, however, the Glastonbury group's members decided to feature only local producers and retailers that sold local food, and to call their publication a directory – decisions that suited them and their intentions for the project.

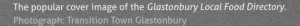

A celebration of local food
A local food guide for Glastonbury and the surrounding area

TRANSITION GLASTONBURY

FIRST EDITION 2008

The popular cover image of the *Glastonbury Local Food Directory*. Photograph: Transition Town Glastonbury

The action

Caroline Lewis helps to coordinate the town's food group, and has also been heavily involved in putting the directory together. Early on in the process, the team held an open consultation meeting about plans for the directory, which gave other local people a feeling of involvement and an opportunity to contribute ideas. A group of volunteers then set about devising a questionnaire and delivering it to the relevant local businesses – and chasing up those that didn't answer questions correctly, or at all! Once the forms were collected, Caroline collated all the information while other volunteers went about drawing up two maps – one of the retailers, another of the producers.

Because this group had a smaller budget than the one in Totnes, it was decided that its members would do all the design and layout themselves (see right for an example of one of their maps) – each person putting in many hours of voluntary time. They did, however, have funding to cover the printing costs, from a £850 grant they received from the Mendip District Council. Half of the businesses featured in the directory donated £10, and together with other funds drawn from the Transition Town Glastonbury purse, and a grant from the organisation Somerset Food Links, there was enough money to print up 5,000 copies of the directory and 1,000 leaflets advertising the launch, and to run the launch itself.

The group focused the launch activities on local children and their families, delivering the leaflets to the schools in the area. On the launch day local celebrity chef Martin Blunos hosted a food trail around the town, which culminated in a prize-giving ceremony for participating children (with prizes donated by local food producers). At the same time, 300 directories were handed out free to people in the town. Following the launch event, more directories

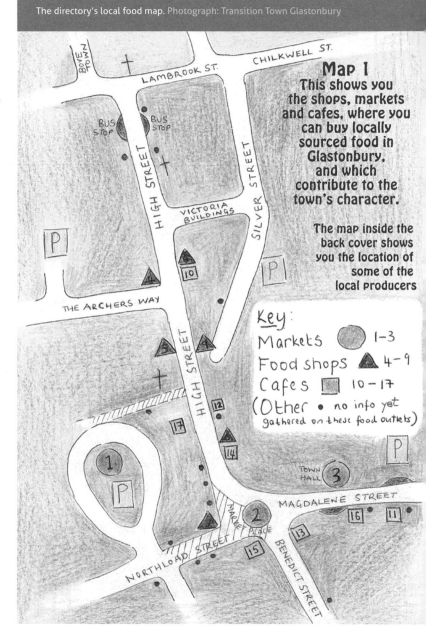

The directory's local food map. Photograph: Transition Town Glastonbury

Map 1 This shows you the shops, markets and cafes, where you can buy locally sourced food in Glastonbury, and which contribute to the town's character.

The map inside the back cover shows you the location of some of the local producers

Key:
Markets ● 1–3
Food shops ▲ 4–9
Cafes ■ 10–17
Other ● no info yet gathered on these food outlets

were distributed through local shops (including hairdressers, pet shops and garages!) and, despite the large number of directories to be shifted, 4,000 were picked up by members of the community in only a few months. Caroline puts the directory's popularity partly down to the fact that many local shops were happy to stock it, and also to the colourful images and artwork that drew many people to the publication. Despite grant delays, the project has therefore grown to be a community success that has stimulated much discussion amongst local businesses and people about the importance of local food and how to go about finding it in the town.

Project name: The Eat Local Resource Guide and Directory

Location: Boulder, Colorado, US

Aim: To develop an online directory of all local food sources and related organisations and businesses throughout the county.

Started: January 2007

How many people involved: Eight volunteers

On the web: www.eatlocalguide.com.
See also www.transitionbouldercounty.org

The idea

The process of producing hard-copy local food directories, made of old-fashioned (and sustainably produced!) paper, is a good way of getting a foot in the door of local businesses, having a local food presence on shop counters, and of generating face-to-face communication around the subject of local food. But once the information has been collected, opening it up to the World Wide Web is a good way of making hard work go even further, and of making future additions and amendments easier and less costly. One place where this has been done to much acclaim is Boulder County, Colorado, in the US.

Boulder is a large county that lies to the north-west of Denver and covers the Rocky Mountain National Park. The organisation Boulder County Going Local had been running for three years before joining the Transition Network and changing its name to Transition Boulder County in early 2008. It thereby became the very first Transition initiative in the US, and Michael Brownlee and other founders have since been at the forefront of Transition activity in their home country. They have also been responsible for sparking a whole range of projects and campaigns, including creating a social networking website (see www.transitioncolorado. ning.com); running permaculture courses; holding many public-awareness events, talks and film screenings; and operating as a hub for other Transition initiatives in their area (it is well worth having a look at their website for inspiration, or simply to be impressed!). An assessment carried out by the organisation found that food sourced from within the county is currently sufficient for only 20,000 of its 300,000 residents. To try to address the 280,000-person shortfall, it has embarked on 'Eat Local, Grow Local, Buy Local' campaigns, all of which are tied together by the online directory.

The directory was inspired by a food map produced in nearby Fort Collins County, but Michael and others soon decided that there were simply too many resources to fit on to a map, and so chose to publish a free booklet containing all local food listings together with articles on local food and agriculture. Unlike the two directories described earlier, Michael and the seven other volunteers working on the Boulder project decided to go for advertiser sponsorship to cover the costs of publication and design, and to use some funds already built up within their own organisation.

The action

Because the team was covering such a vast area, its work was intensive and slow. As with the Glastonbury directory, the folk in Boulder decided to include only those businesses and organisations that dealt with local food in the county. But this led to a number of tangled issues that were hard to unravel, such as finding out for certain whether food outlets do really source local food, and deciding how much would need to be served to qualify them for a place in the directory. The team resolved these issues by asking chefs directly which local producers they used, and also by linking in with the Boulder County Farmers' Market to find out which local restaurants got the producers' thumbs-up.

When all the information was collected and collated, it was written up. Businesses were organised into the following categories: Beef, lamb and poultry, Dairy and eggs, Honey, Wine and mead, Water, Restaurants and caterers, Farmers' markets, Grocers, Gardens, Green-houses and Organisations. Each entry was listed with contact details and a brief description. Twenty-five thousand copies were published and distributed for free through local shops and at Transition events.

But the project did not end there, as the team was keen to make its hard work even more widely available by transferring all the information to a website created for the purpose (www.eatlocalguide.com), together with accompanying sections for local food articles, news and events. A brief look through its mouth-watering array of local food listings is enough to make Boulder County seem like a very attractive place to live and eat!

Some closing thoughts on local food guides and directories

Local food guides and directories, while they can effectively tie together and present the full local food picture in a community, do presuppose the existence of a local food network that is interesting and extensive enough to guide people towards. If that is not yet the case in a particular area, community groups may choose to focus their energies on building it up before researching and listing producers and initiatives within it. But once the time is right and the network is ripe for such a guide, its paper or cyber publication represents a celebration of a community's work and its appreciation of locally grown, locally produced and locally served food.

Tips on compiling local food guides and directories

As suggested by Noni Mackenzie (A Celebration of Local Food), Caroline Lewis (The Glastonbury Local Food Directory) and Michael Brownlee (The Eat Local Resource Guide and Directory).

1. Use a directory project as an opportunity to link in with other relevant organisations and local government bodies in your community, such as the Chamber of Commerce, farmers' markets and regional Food Links organisations.

2. Set yourselves deadlines for when you want information to be collected from businesses, and don't be afraid to nag if necessary.

3. Give businesses clear guidelines on the information you'd like from them (either with standard interview questions or in the form of questionnaires).

4. Chat with business owners face to face – it is the best way of making them feel included and valued by the directory project, and they will then be much more likely to cooperate.

5. Make sure everyone involved in the directory group feels valued – how the directory group operates is very important. Each member will be going into the community as an ambassador of the project, and if individuals feel they have shared ownership over its direction there is more chance that they will present a clear, passionate vision to those they speak with.

6. Persevere! There will likely be times when efforts to include everyone's points of view lead to loggerheaded debates, but working through opposing opinions can throw up some fascinating discussions and even generate creative ideas.

7. Have a core team of at least three people before embarking on the project, and make sure responsibility is distributed according to each person's ability and time availability.

8. It is also important that the group is not dependent on any one member – that it can function well even if the meat-and-fish-shop researcher, for example, has to leave.

9. Take good notes at each meeting and share them with all members.

10. Make sure the final publication is thorough, well researched and as colourful, vibrant and eye-catching as possible – you want local people to be really grabbed by it and sucked into the importance of what it represents!

11. Selling advertising space to fund a directory project can help to favour what are usually the more lucrative local businesses over others. On the other hand, it can be a very helpful boost to the project's funds and can help it go much further while also raising extra money for the wider local food initiative. Which side of the advertising fence you fall on will depend on your own views and those held by fellow group members.

Resources

See page 203 for Local food guides and directories and Local food – general, and page 197 for Funding, grants and loans.

Chapter 12

SCHOOL PROJECTS ON LOCAL FOOD

A poster from Transition Town Kinsale's schools programme.
Photograph: Transition Town Kinsale

EDUCATION FOR SUSTAINABILITY
INSPIRING CARE FOR THE EARTH

Our modern way of life, for all its convenience and luxury, is dependent upon a level of resource consumption which is, in short, unsustainable.

Children are the future. If humankind is to make the vital steps towards a culture of balance, living within the Earth's limited resource base, then it is today's children who are required to learn **skills, perspectives** and **values** which can create and sustain such a future.

Our Involvement in the school can feed into other programs (e.g. 'Green Schools') and into the existing curriculum. We have also devised our own flexible program, as follows:

OUR PROGRAM

Our program includes 3 elements:

1. *Classroom based exploration of aspects of sustainability.* Including;
- **Energy:** How much we need/use. Where it comes from. Renewable/fossil fuels.
- **Materials/Resources:** What we need/use. Where things come from. How things are made.
- **Food:** Global/local. Packaging. Farming/growing practices.
- **Concerns:** Pollution. Climate Change. Resource shortage (e.g. dwindling oil and gas reserves).

These themes will be explored in an open, inclusive, group brainstorm/discussion format. This will encourage children to share their own knowledge, and to realise the many links between the connected aspects involved. Simple, practical solutions will present themselves naturally to young, engaged minds.

2. *Practical Skills.* To suit the preference/requirements/capacities of each school. Options Include:
- **Recycling:** Craft activities to make practical items, gifts, and art.
- **Planting trees:** Native sp. /fruit trees.
- **Creating a garden:** Fruits, vegetables, herbs and flowers. Living willow
- **Making Preserves:** Jam, Pickle, from local produce.
- **Composting:** Setting up a school system.

Our emphasis will be on group work, a fun attitude (e.g. making up funny work songs) and engagement with natural materials. We will encourage the involvement of other teaching staff and parents, in order to ensure the continued benefits of projects in the school grounds.

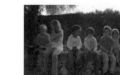

3. *Woodland Visit.* Day of fun activities in a local forest. Featuring:
- **'Earth Walk':** A guided walk, with activities designed to awaken and enrapture each of the different senses.
- **Tree Talk:** A group contemplation of the importance of trees to our existence. Economy, Ecology and Ancient Heritage.
- **Shelter construction:** Making a simple, low impact dwelling.
- **Games:** Running, jumping and playing in our (primal) natural habitat.
A packed lunch picnic, rainproof clothes (just in case) and parent helpers (to make up the adult: child ratio) will all be required.

A school is a social hub where parents, children, cleaners, cooks, administrators and teachers all interact. Because it is such a focus point for community life it is also, in many cases, the perfect venue for effecting food-culture change and for ensuring that transformative ripples are felt far beyond the school gate. Children are of course an important focus for local food awareness in their own right – it is they who will have to cope with the legacies of climate change and of the limits of cheap oil. So in helping them to make connections between food, nature and human health, and to open their eyes to the possibility that they can question and change practices exploiting these connections, we are taking an important step towards undoing the damage we present them with. But we do have some way to go. A survey in 2007 found that one in ten eight-year-olds didn't know where yoghurt comes from, or that pork comes from pigs, while a thankfully smaller 2 per cent of city-based children surveyed thought that eggs come from cows.[1] It is precisely this kind of detachment from the source of their own meals that can foster a disinterest or ignorance in young people of the consequences of mass-produced, centrally distributed, pesticide-heavy and nutritionally empty food.

School food in this country has pulled its nutritional socks up in recent years, and it is hoped that new government nutrition standards will ensure that more of the three million school meals served daily[2] are healthier and freshly prepared. But there is still a large gap between preparing healthy, fresh meals and schools thoroughly supporting a shift in sustainable farming and growing (both through education of their pupils and procurement of their food). Encouraging schools to plan the continual provision of nutritious meals once the fuel tanks run dry is a further step still. But, on a positive note, this does mean that there is much scope for community groups wanting to focus their energies on school work.

Any of the other projects mentioned in this book could potentially be adapted to school participation – children are, after all, as involved in the food supply chain as adults and can contribute to, or at least learn from, every stage within it. They could help plant a new community orchard, design leaflets for a new food co-op, have regular work sessions at a local CSA, be part of a reskilling-for-kids programme, or run a stall at a farmers' market selling their own school produce. The nature of a school project may well be dictated by the availability of skills within your group or among your contacts in the community – especially if you have experienced cooks or gardeners in your midst. And it helps of course if they also know how to inspire respect and a sense of fun in the children they work with. Such was the case in Transition Town Kinsale, where local permaculture students (with experience of working in schools) devised a whole programme of sustainable learning for primary school children, centred around growing, harvesting and cooking up their own school-grown food (see their poster on the previous page).

You may choose to use a school-based project as an opportunity for community engagement, or to form links with organisations that can help facilitate food-focused learning. Involving schoolchildren in food-related projects could also be one way of drawing them into the wider process of food relocalisation, and of giving their own post-peak-oil visions a place and a voice. But, whatever schoolwork you embark upon and however you go about involving the kids, make sure they find it fun.

The following are just three examples of the vast variety of local food-centred projects currently feeding small stomachs and minds in schools around the UK, all of which have taken their first exploratory steps towards building food resilience in their communities.

School project stories

Project name: Naturewise Community Forest Garden

Location: Islington, North London

Aim: To connect inner-city dwellers with nature and its edible bounties.

Started: 1995

How many people involved: Many volunteers, schoolchildren and visitors over the years.

On the web: www.naturewise.org.uk

The idea

Children living in urban centres rarely have the opportunity to engage with food production, or to fully experience the connections between what they eat and the wider natural world. That is, unless they are lucky enough to live near one of the many food-growing or garden projects that are springing up in cities around the world to help counteract concrete desertification (see Chapter 6, Community gardens), or if their school makes space in its curriculum and playground for the children to explore the process of growing food from seeds, and making meals from what they grow.

One unique project in Islington, North London gives children the chance not only to learn about edible growing first hand but also to enjoy it in the context of a wild and beautiful forest garden. Developed by Robert Hart on his Shropshire smallholding in the 1960s, forest gardening is a form of food production that imitates and facilitates the natural growth patterns of a forest. In this system, a diverse variety of edible crops are planted according to the following seven layers: the canopy, the low trees, the shrubs, the herbaceous plants, the ground-cover layer of horizontal plants, the underground root layer and, lastly, the vertical, climbing plants. Beyond the planting phase, this method requires virtually no inputs because it works as a self-sustaining ecosystem, which is why a growing number of forest-garden supporters describe the approach as being well suited to feeding communities in an energy-lean world. Alongside its high levels of energy efficiency, forest gardening can also produce fantastic yields. Another forest garden pioneer, Martin Crawford (see his article on page 99) estimates that one acre of forest garden can produce enough to feed ten people (approximately double what is produced in monocrop agriculture). High yields and efficiency aside, forest gardens are also lush and vibrant places. Being as they are biodiverse nature havens, they could not be further removed from the bland monotony of the vast, single-crop fields that dominate industrial farming.

The action

So the children of Islington are getting a head start in one form of post-oil food production that can feed the belly and the senses besides. Their forest garden, which covers nearly an acre in the grounds of the Margaret Macmillan Nursery School, was designed and planted in 1995 by volunteers working with Naturewise – a community-run permaculture initiative based in the area (see www.naturewise.org.uk) and coordinated under the committed gaze of Alpay Torgut, a permaculture teacher now living in Wales.

As the Margaret Macmillan school follows an ethos of encouraging children to learn through nature, having a living forest garden as an outdoor classroom has given it the ideal setting in which to put its principles into practice. The arrangement is that Naturewise monitors and attends to the upkeep of the site, using it as a venue for workshops, permaculture courses and community work sessions at weekends, while the children play in and learn from the garden during the week. Around them grow apples, pears, grapes, almonds, medlars, hazelnuts, onions, redcurrants and much, much more.

The rewards

The upkeep of the forest garden has ebbed and flowed since its planting over fourteen years ago, but it is now enjoying a resurgent flow under the guidance of Claire White, community gardener at the Spitalfields Housing Cooperative, Naturewise volunteer and permaculture teacher. Claire describes the garden as a valuable learning resource for all the adults and children who use it, because, as an ecosystem made up of beneficial, interconnected relationships, it is a living metaphor for understanding and bringing about cooperation in the human world. Again, this is in contrast to an industrial approach to agriculture that seeks to dominate rather than respect the soil, plants, insects, water and air it also depends upon. Over the years, children and teachers have harvested fruit, berries, nuts and herbs; made compotes and jams; watched the trees grow and the insects thrive; and have learned to recognise plants that are edible and those that can sting. As Claire points out, the garden shows its visitors that land can have multifunctional uses even when it is used as a site for food production – that it can be a place for play, work, learning and inspiring as well as being a source of fresh, local nourishment, which is all the more remarkable considering it is just 3☐ miles away from Trafalgar Square.

Not all schools are fortunate enough to have the space (or the enthusiasm of a nearby group of permaculturalists) that would allow them to establish a fully fledged edible forest. But, as Claire says, the same principles of planting in seven layers can be used in much smaller school, home and community gardens to maximise the use of space, provide a home for wildlife and grow a variety of crops. Because of the timely relevance of the forest-gardening approach, more and more people are learning how to apply its principles and to share their knowledge with others (see Martin Crawford's website www.agroforestry.co.uk for details of related courses, books and DVDs). Forest gardens are particularly appropriate for school settings because they can be designed to include plants and trees that fruit during term-time, and to be relatively maintenance-free in the holidays. But they also have so much going on in them in terms of plant, soil and insect life that they are simply magical places for children to be.

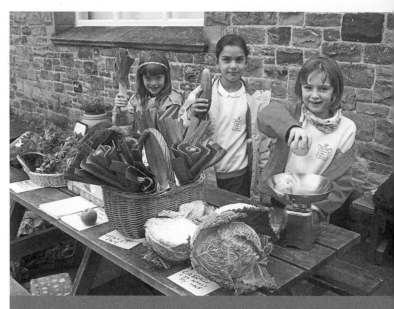

Proud veg stallholders in a Tynedale primary school.
Photograph: Transition Town Tynedale

Project name: The Playground Veg Stall

Location: Tynedale, Northumberland

Aim: To encourage local schoolchildren and their parents to buy local, organic veg.

Started: September 2008

How many people involved: One volunteer organiser, up to twelve children running the stall (three at any one time), many growers from the nearby MENCAP College.

Transition initiative website: www.transitiontynedale.org

If there is no readily available person in your community who can be called upon to deliver a local food programme or set up a forest garden for local children – or if you are looking to supplement such a programme with other school-based activities – there are many ways of engaging teachers and pupils in how to grow, harvest, sell, process, preserve, cook and enjoy local food.

The idea

In the rural district of Tynedale, Northumberland, the local Transition group wanted to find a way of encouraging children to start thinking about where their food comes from, and why it is important to favour local produce. Group members approached the Dilston MENCAP College, where people with disabilities learn to grow and harvest organic produce for their own box scheme. The college agreed to collaborate by providing vegetables for a weekly stall in a school playground. In the meantime Ross Menzies, a Transition Tynedale participant, managed to arrange a weekly playground slot on Wednesday afternoons in his daughter's school.

The rewards

It was not long before the first stall was up and running, and pupils were being given the opportunity to take on stallholding responsibilities. Parents at the school have been buying vegetables that would otherwise have been bought from the supermarket, and some of them have begun to donate surplus produce from their own gardens. It has also been a hit with the college and the Parent-Teacher Association, who are grateful for the extra income they share between them. Ross and others have managed to run the project entirely on volunteer time and with no funding at all. They have been delighted with its success and hope to run it out to other local schools further down the line.

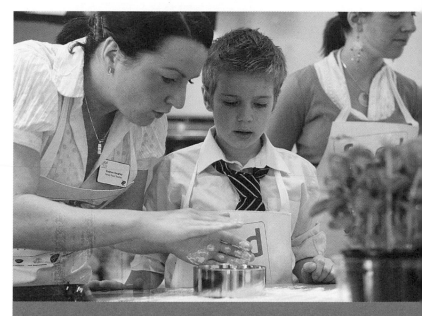

A Food For Life rep cooking with students at Eastwood School, Nottingham. Photograph: Eastwood Comprehensive

Project name: Food For Life

Location: Eastwood Comprehensive School, Nottingham

Aim: To transform the school's food culture, engage the children in food production and involve the wider community in the process.

Started: January 2008

How many people involved: Numerous pupils, teachers, parents and community members.

On the web: www.foodforlife.org

The Food For Life Partnership

By slotting their project into extra-curriculum hours, the folk in Tynedale managed to bring local food issues into the school sphere without impinging on lesson time. Trying to encourage teachers and school managers to make space in their already tightly packed schedules for food-focused learning is not always an easy task. But for community groups hoping to extend local food awareness to children in their area, there is always the option of introducing the idea with the backup and support of an established national programme. Schools might feel more comfortable participating in a project run by experienced experts, and perhaps more amenable to replacing their tarmac and manicured lawns with edible plant life.

The following project is one of many that have been enabled by such a national programme – the Food For Life Partnership. We have included this particular programme here (and there are of course many other community-based, local-food-focused projects out there, being run by charities and non-profit-making organisations across the country) because a number of Transition initiatives have already expressed interest in the scheme. By availing themselves of the expertise, materials and knowledge that organisations such as Food For Life can offer, community groups can take a step back from reinventing more wheels and cut down on their own work time. Because this programme is designed to harness community ideas and input, it is particularly appropriate to the aims of Transition initiatives and other community-engaged local food projects that are focusing their energies around school-based or other forms of public-sector work.

The Lottery-funded Food For Life Partnership, together with its partners the Soil Association, Garden Organic, Focus on Food and the Health Education Trust, works with public-sector caterers, schools and their surrounding communities to help them improve their food culture and incorporate more local and organic food into their meals. In schools, they do this through a number of different approaches: teaching the children how to grow, prepare and cook food, getting the school cooks on board to support a healthier school vision, connecting with local farms, and finally transforming the school's food procurement and menu – all of which are facilitated by skilled representatives from the partner organisations, located in each region of the country.

One of the first stages is to set up a School Nutrition Action Group (SNAG), comprised of pupils, parents and teachers, and community members – the perfect opportunity for local residents to become involved.

The purpose of a SNAG is to create a school food policy and action plan by bringing together the ideas and perspectives of people within and around the school community. Once a plan is in place, local representatives of the Food For Life partner organisations are on hand to get things moving. Participating schools are rewarded with Food For Life standards of bronze, silver or gold, the idea being that they can progress through the standards as their food culture improves. Schools reaching the bronze level have 75 per cent of their meals freshly prepared, have set up a SNAG, and provide opportunities for farm visits, food growing and cooking. When they reach silver, schools have a range of organic, local and free-range foods on their menus, have a cooking club set up where pupils can learn to prepare produce they've grown, and there have been concerted efforts to involve the wider community through events, workshops, etc. On achieving a gold standard, schools will be serving at least 75 per cent freshly prepared, 50 per cent locally sourced and 30 per cent organic food, every pupil in the school has the opportunity to grow and prepare food, and groups of children are actively involved in regular work on a local farm. Some participating schools may of course choose to continue on their healthy path and work to achieve 100 per cent organic and local food to their children – a tall but not impossible order.

Five hundred schools signed up to the scheme in its first six months, with seventy-three of them choosing to be flagship schools committed to achieving the gold standard award. The Food For Life team hopes to enrol 3,600 more schools by 2012. This is a target that community members can help schools to reach by introducing teachers and parents to the scheme, and eventually becoming involved in the food transition they embark upon.

The action

Eastwood's SNAG was set up in January 2008 and is composed of local parents, residents, policemen and governors as well as the students themselves. Including people from the surrounding community is a crucial part of the process, and a way of allowing the transformation of the school's food culture to also spark change beyond the school walls. As part of the SNAG action plan, James persuaded the school's board of governors to provide funds for edible growing in the grounds. Soon after, in March, pupils volunteered to take part in building raised beds, putting in seeds and growing their crops. To assist them in their work, they had the help and advice of Ruth Hepworth, an experienced gardener from the Food For Life partner organisation Garden Organic. Other teachers and SNAG members also pitched in, from the caretaker to the school cook's dad – all eager to be part of this community dig. In the summer of 2008, pupils were able to take their first harvest to the canteen to be used in school meals. Meanwhile, James established a connection with local farm Redgates, which pupils now visit regularly (including helping out in this year's lambing season) and which supplies the canteen with meat and eggs.

Alongside sharpening their growing and farming skills, pupils have been given the chance to cook their produce, with Year 11 children working towards Basic Food Hygiene qualifications, and many others helping to prepare food served at school performances and community events held in school venues. Pupils now play a large role in identifying what changes need to happen in their school's food culture, and in deciding how to go about effecting those changes. They have, for example, chosen what food is grown in the raised beds, decided to source more local food for the school menu, and redecorated the canteen walls.

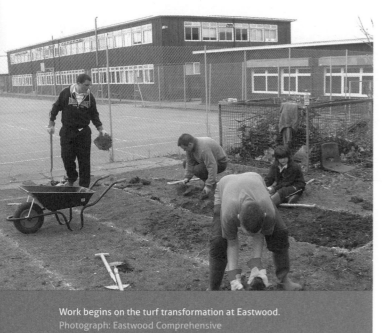

Work begins on the turf transformation at Eastwood.
Photograph: Eastwood Comprehensive

Food For Life at Eastwood Comprehensive: the idea

One of the flagship schools that has radically over-hauled its food culture via the Food For Life programme is Eastwood Comprehensive School in Nottingham. Teacher James Spriggs was inspired to sign his school up having seen the gardener (and Soil Association president) Monty Don's success in working an allotment with a group of disaffected young people. As the Inclusion Unit Manager for Eastwood, a secondary school set in a disadvantaged area, James thought the programme would be a great way of engaging all pupils – from the less-enthusiastic to the gifted learners – through the medium of good food, and getting tastier, healthier school meals on plates in the process.

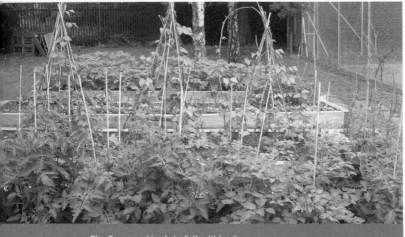

The Eastwood beds in full edible glory.
Photograph: Eastwood Comprehensive

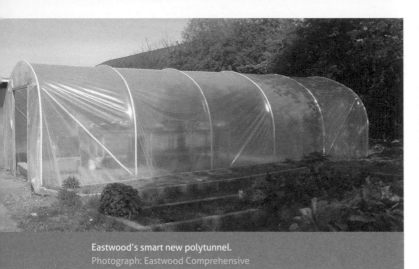

Eastwood's smart new polytunnel.
Photograph: Eastwood Comprehensive

The rewards

James points out that not only are the students much happier with the food they eat at school, but they have also enjoyed boosts to their confidence and a sense of pride over the food-based work they've been a part of. Awareness of food, from where and how it is grown to how it is eaten and enjoyed, is now a central and growing part of Eastwood and the community beyond its grounds. This year, the school received planning permission to put up a 30-foot polytunnel to extend the growing season, which, at the time of writing, has just been erected. The hope and aim is to provide the school canteen with salad and vegetables all year round. James has also had reports of a number of parents, students and staff starting to grow food in their gardens, which just goes to show how infectious growing-enthusiasm can be, and how nurturing schoolchildren to be green-fingered diggers can have a profound and far-reaching effect on the wider community's relationship to food.

Tips on running local food projects in schools

As suggested by Claire White (Naturewise Community Forest Garden), Ross Menzies (The Playground Veg Stall) and James Spriggs (Food For Life Partnership, Eastwood Comprehensive School).

1. If you have a particular school in mind, assess its willingness to participate in a food project by chatting with the relevant teachers and, at the same time, work on galvanizing support amongst parents. It might then be a good idea to hold an initial brainstorming session between parents, teachers, pupils and, if appropriate, other community members, to look at options and possible plans (i.e. whether you want to start with a small extra-curricular activity, to work on a growing project with the help of local permaculturalists or gardeners, or sign up for a long-term

programme such as that offered by Food For Life – or do something else!).

2. Ensure that the children's safety is protected at all times, and that the project is carried out in accordance with the school's own rules. This will mean in many cases running Criminal Record Bureau (CRB) checks on any non-teacher adults partaking in the work, making sure children are given proper guidance in whatever task they're doing, overseeing all potentially hazardous work (with knives, pitchforks, hammers, etc!) and, if necessary, taking out insurance for project facilitators.

3. Don't overload the teachers. On the whole, ideas that entail little time or input from busy teachers will be the most popular with participating schools. This means the onus needs to fall on parents, external facilitators or other community members to take the bulk of the project on.

4. Keeping good communication channels open between project organisers and teachers is crucial. Make sure the teachers and the school as a whole are clear about what they are taking on, what is expected of them, and the direction the project hopes to take.

5. Use the project as a springboard for exploring other environmental issues by holding related events, doing food-themed drama or art projects, and running games sessions (see books in the Resources section for imaginative eco-games from the field of environmental education and forest schooling.)

6. Don't let your own inexperience in food growing hold you back, whether you are a teacher or community member. If you ask for help and assistance from others within or beyond the school, you may well find what you need.

7. If planting in the school grounds, go for plants that are popular with children, such as berry bushes or blossoming fruit trees.

8. Keep in mind that, ideally, you want to be harvesting as much produce as possible during term time, so try to focus on plants whose fruits will mature before the summer holidays arrive.

9. As mentioned earlier, whatever shape or form the project takes on, keep it fun.

Resources

See page 207 for School projects on local food, page 200 for General edible gardening and page 197 for Funding, grants and loans.

Chapter 13

LOCAL FOOD EVENTS

FOOD FOR THOUGHT
an evening dedicated to food

presented by Transition Town West Kirby

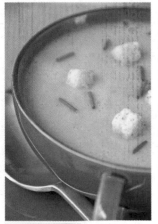

Looking at the benefits of eating locally grown seasonal food – for the community, the environment and our taste buds!

Plus ...

Why food prices are rising and how Transition Towns are leading the way in promoting local food provision.

food to taste on the night!

speakers include:
Ken Dowden on simple ways to grow your own food, Church Farm Organics Ltd, Claremont Farm and La Paz restaurant (Wirral Chef of the Year 2007).

Wednesday 23 January at 7.30pm
URC, Meols Drive, West Kirby CH48 5DA (200m from train station)
All Welcome – Admission Free – Donations Welcome
www.transitiontowns.org/West-Kirby

CLAREMONT FARM

'Local food events' is nearly as broad a category as food itself, but we have included it here because one-off, or regular but infrequent events of this kind can provide a valuable opportunity for groups to hoist up and wave the local food flag within a community. Because they are rarer happenings than, say, weekly markets or co-op collections, they can be energetic hubs within a community's social calendar, helping to sharpen focus on the issues they present and showcase local food work happening nearby. The local food events described here have awareness raising as their central aim – but spinning off from that can be many other positive consequences for a local food network, from facilitating communication between producers to engaging the community in food-production activities. Depending on their focus, they can provide space for home-growers to find kindred green-fingered spirits, community orchards to press and sell their juice, consumers to sample local cheeses or CSAs to recruit new members. Tying the activities together under one themed banner helps to grab public attention, whether that theme is based on the seasonal produce of the time (such as an Apple Day, a Berry Celebration, or a general Harvest Festival), a particular focus of food production (as in a 'Grow Your Own' day or a Seed Swapping event), the local food initiatives and producers themselves (such as a 'Meet Your Local Farmers' day), or some kind of community activity (as in a local food treasure hunt or a picnic on a community farm).

Apart from choosing an eye-grabbing theme, other key factors that help determine the success of a local food event include the following.

- When it is held. Plan to hold it at a time, day and date that works for the kind of people you're aiming at, and that doesn't clash with other community events.

- Where it is held. A prominent venue is preferable, but if one is not available, attention-drawing posters and bunting can make up for that. Choosing a venue that has the necessary facilities (such as kitchens, toilets, stages, etc.) is another obvious but important consideration.

- How it is publicised. Using the normal PR routes can be done in a creative, witty way, or there's always the option of teaming up with local musicians or artists to come up with some colourful publicity stunts.

- Lastly, what it is! Making it fun and enticing, from its title to its activities, is key. Keep in mind, for instance, that including entertainment and activities for children will help to draw in the parents, and having local food available will help to draw in anyone with a healthy appetite.

Because local food events do not necessarily require ongoing commitment, they can be relatively easy projects to get off the ground and good starting places for community groups wanting to galvanize their neighbours into local food action. And, perhaps for this reason, the young Transition movement has already played host to a vibrant variety of local food events in the past couple of years, from the small to the large, and the simple to the ambitious. The following are some examples of these events.

Local food event stories

Project name: The Nottingham Urban Harvest Festival

Location: Nottingham

Aim: To hold a secular harvest celebration in the city to promote local food while also drawing existing local eco groups and food groups together under the Transition umbrella.

Held: 5 October 2008

How many people involved: Five organisers, approximately 900 participants.

Transition initiative website: www.transitionnottingham.org.uk

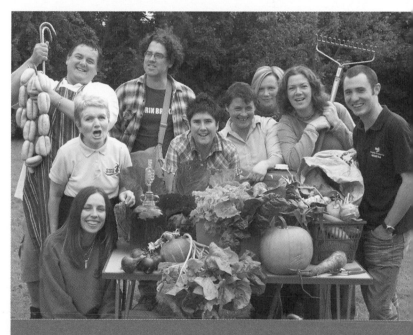

The Urban Harvest Festival organisers.
Photograph: Transition City Nottingham

The idea

Despite the grumbles of sceptics and the best efforts of the English weather, the following was a large and ambitious event that became a huge success. In July 2008 Clare Davies, a local permaculture designer, came home after a Transition City Nottingham meeting and, feeling frustrated with what she saw as an imbalance of too much talk and not enough action within the group, determined to give one of her ideas some proactive shape. Her plan was to hold a harvest festival within the city, and she sat down to explore the idea in a mind map. Clare later took her mind map to the steering group, who deemed it too big, complicated and impossible a project to pull together within the space of a few months. But Clare was not deterred. She persuaded four others to help her realise her festival vision (none of whom had experience in putting on large-scale events, but all of whom were motivated enough to make their first one work), and they held their first meeting a few weeks later at the beginning of August.

The action

The first task was to find an appropriate venue. After exploring a few options, the group settled on Green's Windmill, a council-owned working windmill near the city centre. The managers there were hugely enthusiastic about the festival idea, which they felt mirrored their own principles of sustainability and community resilience, so they happily offered the site to Clare and company at a drastically reduced rate.

The next stage was to recruit stallholders for the event, which was simply a matter of trawling the shops and markets of Nottingham, chatting to producers and business owners (as well as contacts they passed on) and trying to get them on board. On the whole, the responses they received were enthusiastic – so much so

that the few reluctant contacts could be left unpursued without much dent in the total number of stall participants. The event also attracted enough participating businesses and projects for the team to be able to be quite strict about including only those that were from within the city – one willing organic box scheme was turned down because it was located too far away.

On the morning of 5 October, the heavens opened and hopes of holding an outdoor bread-making workshop were dashed. But rain (and the odd technical hitch) aside, the rest of the event went according to plan and the public turned up in full force. The festival was organised into zones, including the barter, market, music and information zones. There were also numerous activities and workshops going on throughout the day, including film screenings, an interactive map and apple pressing run by the folk from St Ann's Allotments (as described on pages 65-8) – the latter being so popular that they eventually ran out of apples. Other stalls included a local butcher, a wine circle, a box scheme, vegan cakes and of course Transition City Nottingham.

The success of this event is particularly remarkable considering it was run on only £145 that Clare made by rattling her old biscuit tin among local groups. This money was put together with the £10 paid by each stallholder, and used to cover the site rent and other materials and equipment for the day. All the organisers worked voluntarily (the web design and development alone would have otherwise cost around £3,000), and much of the promotion was done via word of mouth. The website created to advertise the event proved to be an invaluable promotional tool, and it was soon picked up by Google. The team posted a downloadable poster and flyer on the site that interested locals could print off and put up themselves. Local media helped spread the story, and interviews with Clare were in local papers and on BBC Nottingham radio shows.

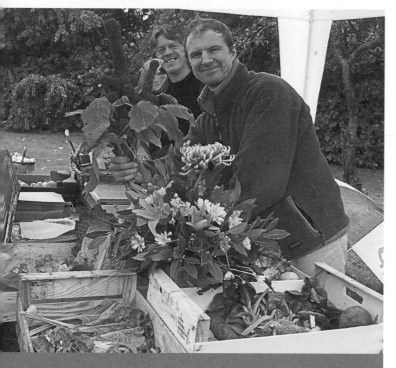

Trinity Farm's stall at Nottingham's Urban Harvest Festival.
Photograph: Transition City Nottingham

The rewards

Clare noticed much networking between stallholders, and is convinced that the event played an important role in helping to strengthen the local food network within Nottingham. She also thinks that many people came along because of a love of food but left with a new awareness of Transition and the power of community action. The events team itself made a number of helpful links through its work on the Harvest Festival, including those with the council's sustainability officers, the Green's Windmill team, the low-carbon transport group The Big Wheel, the horticultural department of Nottingham Trent University and the local tourist board – all of whom hope to collaborate with the team on future projects and events. Clare attributes this flurry of enthusiasm for the team's work to the fact that she and the others were determined to ensure that every connection made was to the mutual satisfaction of both parties – as far as possible, the needs of stallholders, workshop leaders, venue managers and the events team itself were met. So it is no surprise that all stall and workshop participants have agreed to be part of the next Urban Harvest Festival that Clare and team have already been asked to organise – an event preceded by the Great Spring Seed Sowing day in March 2009, where people learned how to sow, grow and harvest edible seeds ready to share their bountiful produce at the Harvest Festival in October.

The Urban Harvest Festival story is one of sheer determination – a heartening example of a small idea that, with vision and much group energy, grew to a large event bringing many city residents closer to local food and the people that produce it.

Project name: Harvest Inspiration

Location: Leicester

Aim: To inspire local people to grow their own fruit and veg, and to draw attention to Transition City Leicester, its food group and its community aims.

Held: 11 October, 2008

How many people involved: Eight volunteer organisers, approximately sixty participants.

Transition initiative website: www.transitiontowns.org/Leicester

The ideas

In a city not too far away from Nottingham and at a time just before Clare Davies' festival vision emerged, Lisa Michael and other Transition City Leicester (TCL) participants were busy drawing themselves together to form the TCL food group. In some of their early discussions in June 2008, a number of group members supported the idea of working on a project to provide novice food growers with the help and advice they needed – something that would encourage others to embark on the home-growing adventure. They came up with a plan to hold a one-off grow-your-own food event in the city centre, and quickly got to work.

The action

The venue they chose was the foyer of a prominent city-centre church (with a rain-proof roof!), and they began raising funds by running a local food cafe in the same place (with cakes, savouries, teas and coffee donated by food group members). This also helped to raise the group's profile, especially as it provided a wonderful spread that was said by one customer to be "the best food to be had in Leicester".

The TCL food group promoted its event by sending press releases to local papers, and by printing up many posters and fliers and putting them up in windows and public noticeboards around the city. But Lisa found that many people were spontaneously drawn to the event on the day because of the banners, the leaflet-givers and the conspicuous apple press that enticed them into the venue.

The array of events and activities on the day included an advice stall for growers run by the Leicester Organic Group; a storytelling corner run by the Leicester Guild of Storytellers; a large display of home-grown produce, from pumpkins to jams, wines to herbal tinctures; a crowd-pleasing apple press; a 'connections' table where people could find details of relevant courses, workshops, allotment sites and Transition events; and of course the popular food group cafe.

The organising team felt theirs was a job well done, and during the course of the event funds were raised, mailing lists extended and networks grown. Lisa proudly recalls one young couple who came along hoping to find a local veg box supplier and who ended up leaving with information on how to grow their own. The gardeners giving advice were in fact amazed at how little some people knew about food growing – which only confirmed the need for an event to promote it. Lisa's only regret was that they hadn't fully clarified their expectations to the participating groups, and, were others not on hand to step in, the odd hole would have been left in the event. But as it was, there were enough hands to help out and fill in, and all in all the day was a resounding success.

Project name: The Growing Local Conference

Location: Bungay, Suffolk

Aim: To provide a space for learning and discussion about local food issues, and to inspire local action around food.

Held: 8 November 2008

How many people involved: Fifteen volunteer organisers, five speakers, approximately 100 participants.

Transition initiative website: www.transitiontowns.org/Bungay

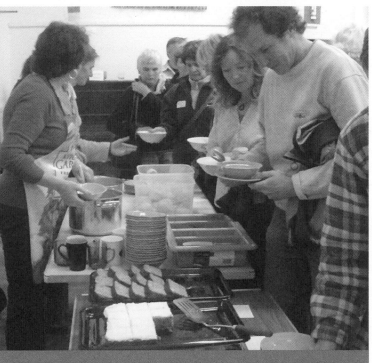

Conference participants enjoying their local lunch.
Photograph: Sustainable Bungay

The idea

This local food event was held in the small market town of Bungay, on the Norfolk–Suffolk border. There, the group known as Sustainable Bungay was formed in November 2007, joining the Transition Network some months later. While the town is fortunate to have a good range of small, independent shops (most likely because they also have no large supermarket), the Sustainable Bungay team is keen to preserve the existing local economy, whilst encouraging a greater shift towards food production in and around the town. So it came up with the idea of holding a local food conference in Bungay to generate awareness and kick-start ideas. A

similar event held the previous year had been a great success and had led to the establishment of Sustainable Bungay – so the team had high hopes for what a local food conference might be able to achieve.

The action

When choosing which speakers to invite to the event, Sustainable Bungay made the most of its contacts within the local food world. One of the team's members, Josiah Meldrum, works for the organisation East Anglia Food Links (see www.eafl.org.uk) and has in the past been involved with community growing projects such as Fordhall Farm and Organic Lea, so was well placed to source an inspirational mix of speakers representing a spectrum of local food work.

The local Methodist church in Bungay had already decided to focus on environmental issues, so was thrilled to be able to host Sustainable Bungay's conference in its hall. This proved to be a mutually beneficial partnership, with members of the congregation promoting, attending and helping to run the event, and the church being enthusiastic about engaging with a wider section of the community.

Beyond the church's assistance in advertising the event, the Sustainable Bungay team also put up posters, gave interviews on local radio, posted the event on every relevant chatroom, blog and website, chatted with other local people, and badgered the local press. News of the event met with much enthusiasm from local residents, with eighty-three people registering beforehand and even more turning up on the day.

The event ran from morning to afternoon, with a free, local, organic meal served at lunchtime. Speakers included Tully Wakeman (the coordinator of East Anglia Food Links and participant of Transition City Norwich), Doeke Dobma (from the National Care

Farming Initiative) and Ru Litherland (the head gardener at Growing Communities, described in detail on page 158-63). The last part of the day was dedicated to an Open-Space-style discussion, where everyone broke off into groups focused on gardens, allotments, farms and public spaces respectively. A number of new ideas and projects emerged from these discussions, including a new garden share scheme, the possibility of setting up a local CSA, the suggestion of initiating a community growing network across East Anglia, and the emergence of a new Transition initiative in the town of Beccles (as well as some Transition mulling over in nearby Lowestoft). At the end of the event a seed swap was held.

All the speakers gave their time for free, but the Sustainable Bungay team covered their travel expenses. Together with the other costs of venue hire, promotion and event materials, the team spent £250 in total out of its members' own pockets. But it managed to raise the same amount through donations from conference participants, and, impressed with Sustainable Bungay's efforts, Suffolk County Council donated a further £250 that will allow the team to put on another event in the future.

Some closing thoughts on local food events

The local food events described in this chapter all required time, effort and group energy to make them happen, but if you have any or all of these inputs in small amounts, then you may want to scale down your aims rather than putting on no such event at all. Below is a short list of a few other ideas to help you conjure up your own.

Other ideas for local food events

- Wild food foraging and feasts.
- Roving local dinner parties in residents' homes.
- Treasure hunts on local farms or in local shops.
- A local food day held jointly between local restaurants.
- A food-waste awareness day.

Tips on holding a local food event

As suggested by Clare Davies (Nottingham Urban Harvest Festival), Lisa Michael (Harvest Inspiration) and Josiah Meldrum (Growing Local Conference).

1. Make sure that the expectation of all organisers is clear from the outset – that they know they're expected to be doers and not just talkers.

2. The pros of having a short lead-up time to organise an event are that the process can be dynamic and exciting – which suits procrastinating types well. But the advantages of having a longer lead-up period are that there is more planning time, there is space to look for sponsors and develop creative ideas, and there is hopefully less stress involved!

3. Cheekiness and determination can go a long way if backed by a strong vision.

4. Don't underestimate how generously people will be prepared to give (time, money, materials, etc.) to such an event – there is much untapped support for local food out there just waiting to be grabbed.

5. It's possible to strike a balance between being realistic and ambitious. If you have a strong conviction that your vision can happen, try not to be pulled down by others whose levels of motivation don't match your own. Having the support of just a few committed others can help to keep the vision alive.

6. Try not to panic on the day if all doesn't go to plan. This is of course easier said than done, but console yourself with the knowledge that unpredictable events can be wonderful opportunities for flexibility and creativity!

7. Remember that free (local, organic) food is a fantastic crowd-pleaser and there are few events that wouldn't benefit from having it on offer.

Resources

See page 203 for Local food events and page 197 for Funding, grants and loans.

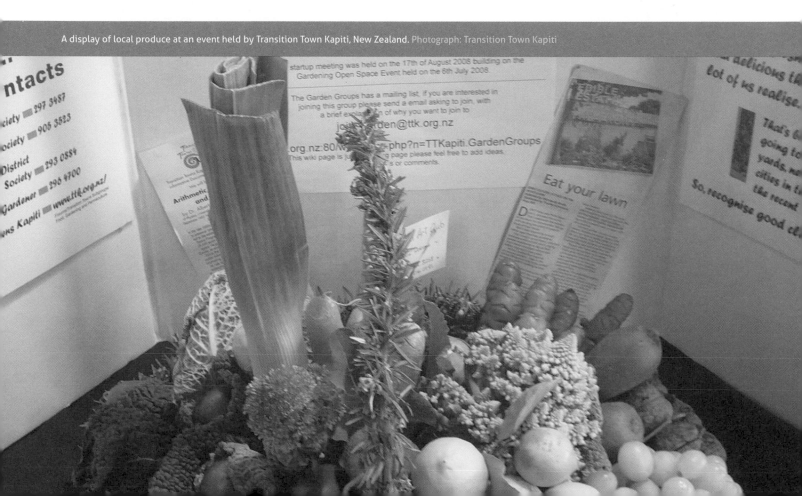

A display of local produce at an event held by Transition Town Kapiti, New Zealand. Photograph: Transition Town Kapiti

Chapter 14

EXPANDING LOCAL FOOD PROJECTS

Successful projects run by passionate local food supporters often end up being widened beyond their original aims. This is done by inspiring and/or helping similar initiatives to set up, by expanding the scope of their own work, by group members developing other, related ideas, or all of the above. A number of these projects also go on to form working relationships with other relevant organisations and initiatives in their areas – local food ventures are twice as likely to collaborate with other businesses than are nationalised food enterprises.[1] Whether or not this was part of the original plan, the need for growth in the local food sector is so strong that when such a project is initiated the many other gaps in food production, processing and supply chains in a given local area become apparent. And once a community group has demonstrated its ability to shape and determine some aspect of its own local food network, it may well have the necessary confidence to go ahead and fill in these gaps. In the meantime, projects may gain enough momentum, attention and support to pull in new blood, and to harness the new energy that will keep the local food ball rolling on.

This chapter features one urban initiative that has drawn a number of local food approaches into its fold, and in so doing has become an integrated model for supplying communities with affordable, organic food produced through small-scale means. As such, it is a model that can be imitated or moulded for application to other community settings, and is well suited to the aims of villages, towns and cities embarking on a transition to greater food resilience.

The Growing Communities story

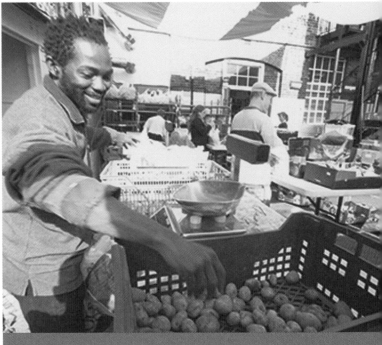

Busy at work in the Growing Communities bag-packing yard.
Photograph: Growing Communities

Project name: Growing Communities

Location: Hackney, London

Aim: To build a community-engaged system of sustainable food trade and production.

Started: 1996

How many people involved: Eight management committee members, eighteen part-time paid members of staff, and up to eighty volunteers in any one year.

On the web: www.growingcommunities.org

The idea

Back in 1996, a group of Hackney residents set out to try to reclaim food production and supply from a system they saw as being environmentally damaging, precarious and contributing to ill health and social breakdown in the communities depending upon it. Together, and on the back of an existing CSA/box scheme they had set up three years before, they formed the aptly named local food initiative Growing Communities, registering as a non-profit-making company limited by guarantee in 1997. One of the founding members was Julie Brown, who is now the organisation's director and who has received much attention and acclaim for her work as a leading social entrepreneur. The Old Fire Station in Hackney, North London is the group's headquarters, and it has established itself as a social enterprise successfully bringing producers closer to the consumers they feed through a number of community-led trading projects. In so doing, Growing Communities has purposely avoided following the example of large-scale, centralised food businesses that exacerbate food insecurities. Instead it has explored and reviewed different ways of sourcing, growing and trading food to develop an alternative way of feeding its urban community.

Central to the group's aims, from the initiative's early beginnings, has been a determination to create a replicable model that other communities can draw from and apply to their own settings.

The way it works

There are three main focuses within the Growing Communities project: trading systems, urban food production and outreach work.

Trading systems

At the level of trading, Growing Communities provides several key outlets for the producers it has formed working relationships with. There is the weekly organic box scheme (the first of its kind in London and actually now a recycled bag scheme), which supplies different-sized selections of fruit and vegetables, delivered by bike or electric milkfloat to one of seven drop-off points in the area. The produce is sourced as locally as possible and supplemented with fruit and veg from sustainable, non-airfreighted sources more further afield. Last year, over 80 per cent of the veg came from the UK, and bananas were the only product brought in from beyond European shores, (see the diagram on page 16, showing what proportion of food is sourced from each 'zone' – the urban domestic, the urban traded, the peri-urban, the rural hinterland, the rest of the UK, the rest of Europe and beyond). Then there is the weekly Stoke Newington Farmers' Market – the only weekly farmers' market in the UK to sell exclusively organic, biodynamic or wild products, and where consumers can buy directly from twenty-two producers, the majority of whom come from within 56 miles of Hackney. There is a large variety of products on offer here, from locally made Turkish pancakes to organic wines; buffalo cheeses to fresh fish; and the market is an important source of income, support and community interaction for the producers that frequent it.

The box scheme and the farmers' market are the two main trading outlets that Growing Communities facilitates, but the project has also encouraged local people to share and exchange their own home-made produce at Good Food Swap events. The main aim of the trading systems as a whole is to harness the buying power of the community and to direct it to the farmers and growers who are producing food in a sustainable way. It is this community-led trade that Growing Communities sees as actively creating the changes it wants to see in the food world.

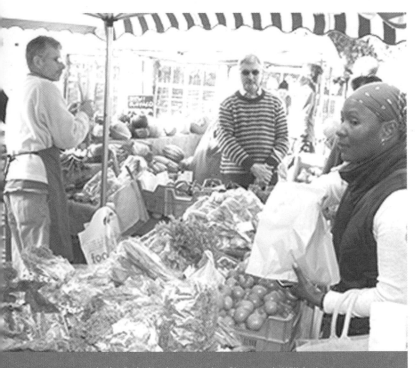

At the Stoke Newington market. Photograph: Will Anderson

Urban food production

Growing Communities' second focus is on urban food production, run from its three organically certified market gardens in Hackney, which specialise in growing mixed salad leaves. Having experimented with different combinations of various crops, they have found salad growing to be the most effective way of providing fresh, local produce all year round, as well as being the most economically viable use of their growing space. It also makes more sense for Growing Communities to grow mixed salads in its own gardens, since the leaves are highly perishable and would not retain as much of their nutritional value if hauled over longer distances. The salads are sold in bags through the box scheme, and the project hopes to be able to supply all of the scheme's salad needs in the near future.

Beyond its market garden work, Growing Communities has helped to plant and set up two nearby community orchards that will provide plums, cherries, hazelnuts, medlars and apples for local people. It has recently established a new Patchwork Farm Project, which is made up of small 'micro-sites' in and around Hackney, and it is also now developing a new Starter Farm Project of larger plots in the peri-urban area around London. A number of Growing Communities 'apprentices' are responsible for growing salad crops on these sites for distribution through the box scheme. All of these projects are innovative ways of bringing farming back into city centres, and together have the potential for drastically increasing the amount of local food accessible to city dwellers.

Outreach work

Though it now has its fingers in many pies, Growing Communities, as its name suggests, is very much embedded in community life – not only through its trading projects but also through its outreach work, the third focus of its time. Part of the philosophy behind actively encouraging community involvement is a perception of the community sphere as being the place where real, effective change can happen – and by teaching, inspiring, training and sharing its work with other community members, the project hopes to spread an appetite for change far and wide. So, aside from channelling the buying power of its community through the box scheme and the market, there are a number of other ways in which Growing Communities pulls community participation into its bag-packing yard and over its garden walls.

At the time of writing, the main focus of the outreach work is to share their business model with others keen to set up similar initiatives. The aim is to enable these groups to initiate their own community-led trading projects to relocalise the local food economy in their areas. In February 2009 the first workshop was held to start the process of mentoring new, Growing-Communities-modelled projects to fruition – an event that was attended by groups from across the UK. The project also shares its work and philosophy with residents in its area through running volunteer schemes, hosting school visits (with garden tours and growing activities for the children) and participating in Food For Life programmes (see page 145) with nearby schools. Local volunteers are in fact a key part of the Growing Communities on-site team, and they can get involved in regular sessions where they learn to sow, grow and harvest food in the gardens alongside Growing Communities growers.

The philosophy

Since the 1990s, Growing Communities has expanded its workforce (to eighteen part-time employees and up to eighty volunteers in a year) and has built up relationships with more farmers and growers (it now works with around twenty-seven local, organic producers). But, despite its growth, it has stayed true to its transparent, participative and community-centred approach. There is, for example, a voluntary management committee that has overall responsibility for the organisation and is elected by and made up of box-scheme members (all of whom are automatically members of Growing Communities itself). The project also makes sure that full details of its accounts are publicly available so that members can see exactly how funds are spent. Although it has been supported by grants from external bodies in the past, the aim has always been that all Growing Communities' core projects be financially independent, and since 2005 100 per cent of its total income has indeed been self-generated. Economic viability is necessary if the project is to remain as a resilient food-trading system for years to come, and as a sustainable model for food supply in other communities.

Julie and others have devised a set of principles guiding Growing Communities' work that help to summarise their aims and focuses described above. Briefly, they describe sustainable food as being:

- ecologically produced (using organic or biodynamic principles, harvested from the wild, or home-grown without the use of artificial pesticides and fertilisers)

- sourced as locally as practicable

- seasonal (so that food seasonal in the UK is prioritised over what is not)

- mainly plant-based (thereby encouraging a reduction in livestock farming)

- fresh or minimally processed

- sourced from small-scale producers.

They aim to distribute their food in a way that:

- supports fair trade (i.e. direct, ongoing communication, fair prices and cooperation with the producers they work with in the UK and abroad)

- involves environmentally friendly practices (with reduced packaging, waste and use of fossil fuels)

- shares knowledge

- fosters community

- strives to be economically viable

- promotes trust through the food chain.

These principles are not rigid or written in stone, but, as Julie points out, they are very much a work in

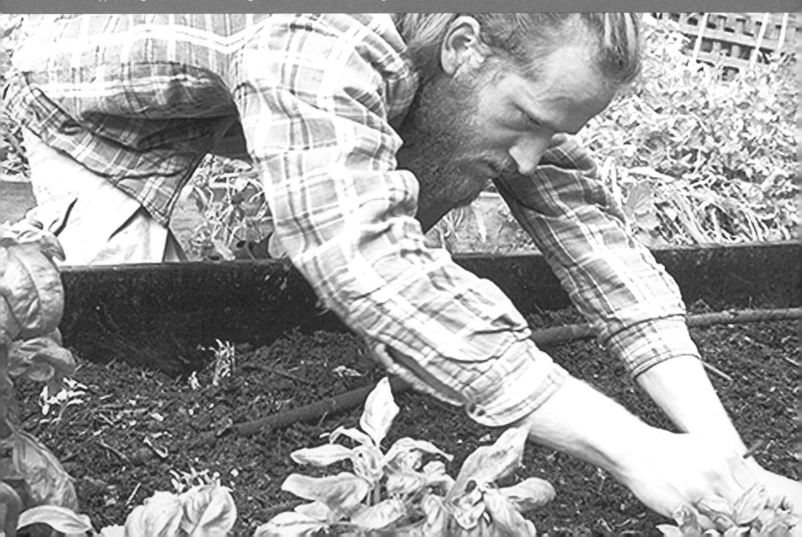

Apprentice grower Sean Hearn tending the basil on one of the Growing Communities micro-sites. Photograph: Growing Communities

progress and can be adapted according to changes that occur within the organisation or the context it is part of. Instead of working to satisfy a consumer desire for cheap and limitless choice, Growing Communities sees its principles as the starting point for deciding what diet we are to follow; what food we are to grow, produce and buy; and what distribution models we are to use. What results is a model that creates and upholds respect for everyone and everything participating in it: farmers, growers, pickers, packers, consumers, eaters and the planet we all live on.

Tips on setting up an initiative based on the Growing Communities model

As suggested by Kerry Rankine (farmers' market organiser at Growing Communities).

1. As the Growing Communities team has found, starting a community-led box scheme is a good first step to relocalising your food supply. It will allow you to get your own produce out to more people while providing a vital outlet for small growers and farmers in your community. It is also something that can work whether you are in an urban or a rural area. You don't need a huge amount of capital or assets to get it going, but you do need some space (for packing and storage) and some helpers.

2. People are the key to making your project work: you need those who really want to make something happen and who are happy to put in a lot of hard work!

3. Think hard about who your customers will be and whether there are people in your area who will want what you are selling!

4. Consider how you are going to communicate what's different or important about what you are doing or selling.

5. Check out the Growing Communities' website (www.growingcommunities.org). It's full of useful information and will continue to be updated with new ideas for helping other community projects to grow.

Resources

See page 195 for Expanding local food projects and page 197 for Funding, grants and loans.

Chapter 15

YET MORE INSPIRED IDEAS

In this chapter we look at further ideas for projects on local food that community groups can get involved in. Some are well-established ideas, while others are newer additions to the local food scene. While many are yet to feature in the local food movement as widely as those described in earlier chapters, they could potentially play an important role in the transition to food resilience.

Community composting

According to Defra, no less than 11.6 million tonnes of biodegradable municipal waste (which includes household food waste) was sent to UK landfills between 2006 and 2007.[1] Not only is it a terrible waste to discard and bury all the nutrients in this organic matter, which might otherwise be used to nourish new plant growth or generate energy, but this waste, once it is in landfill, decomposes and helps to produce the greenhouse gas methane. Under EU law the UK must reduce the amount of biodegradable waste it sends to landfills to 6.3 tonnes by 2013 – and the indications are that the volume is steadily decreasing, as more councils have started up compost-collection schemes and more households are composting at home. By far the most energy-efficient way of eliminating 'compost miles' is to compost your own organic waste and make use of the nutrients within it by using the compost to nourish the soil and edible plants in your own garden. Even if there is a council collection scheme in your area, it is worth finding out where the stuff is taken and ensuring that it is not transported far away before assuming it is a sensible option.

For those who want to find an alternative to council waste-collection schemes, who don't have the outdoor space necessary for composting their biodegradable waste, or who don't produce enough of it or grow enough to make composting a viable thing to do, setting up a community composting scheme can be a good plan. Through such a scheme, waste can be made available, by sale or donation, for other growing projects – to farmers and gardeners who would appreciate and use it. These projects range in scale from residents in a block of flats running a compost site in their grounds, to town-wide collection schemes run alongside vegetable-box deliveries. They could potentially generate income that could be used for other food projects, or be run informally by volunteers keen to get their hands on the soil food lurking in local kitchen bins. Whatever scale, shape and scope it takes on, a community composting scheme could potentially be an important cog in a local food network, making sure a community's organic waste doesn't go to waste.

Resources

See page 191 for Community composting.

Community shops

In the same vein as community orchards or CSAs, community shops are about local people becoming involved in the ownership, decision-making and often the running of a shop in their area. With many small, independent retailers struggling to cope in these credit-crunching times, the idea of community-owned shops is gaining momentum nationwide, with a recent *Guardian* article describing it as "the fast expanding world of the non-profit-making community buyout".[2]

At the time of writing the Rural Community Shops Association, run by the Plunkett Foundation, has 201 community shops listed in its directory, with four new ones added in March 2009 alone. The growing popularity of these shops is testament to the value they have for their surrounding communities. They help to cut down transportation costs and pollution for nearby residents, they are often an important part of the local economy, and they can be thriving social centres where neighbours meet and local events and ads are posted. When shops are taken over by community groups, members can have a say in what is sold, voluntary and paid workers can develop new skills in running the venture, cheaper rates for the premises can sometimes be secured (especially if sited in an existing community building such as a church hall), and once the community has a vested interest in its success there is a greater chance of ensuring the shop's survival. For groups in rural areas interested in saving and/or supporting their shop through community ownership, the Rural Community Shops Association is a good first port of call. It is able to support such ventures with advice and guidance on every stage of the community-ownership process (including finding funding) and has successfully helped many community shops open and thrive over the years. For urban groups wanting to do the same, the organisation Cooperatives UK can provide the necessary assistance.

While there are many community shops around the country supporting their communities in non-grocery ways (as post offices, newsagents, etc.), they can be set up to provide food for local residents and, more specifically, local, organic food sourced directly from nearby producers – thereby giving an extra boost to their local economy. In the UK, two-thirds of all retail food sales are controlled by just four major supermarket chains,[3] and while the shift to local is working to dent these monopolies, community shops could play an important role in reclaiming more of that territory and bringing grocery shopping back to the local community. Community shops are, of course, ideal outlets for selling local produce, helping to shorten food supply chains and extending the community spirit to the farmers and growers in the area. The number of community shops actively working to engage with local producers is growing, and they can be found across the country – from Metfield in Suffolk to the small island of Papa Westray in Scotland. The Making Local Food Work programme, run by an alliance of many local food organisations led by the Plunkett Foundation, is piloting the Community Shops and Local Food project to assess what help these shops need in sourcing produce within a 30-mile radius, in dealing with the producers, and in promoting and selling the food. It then aims to roll out local food toolkits for use in community shops across the UK.

Resources

See page 193 for Community shops.

Food and land mapping

A number of the projects looked at in this book (such as the Open Orchard Project on page 97 and the Glastonbury Local Food Directory on page 136) have engaged in mapping exercises to help further their food-networking aims, but food and land mapping projects are also of great importance in their own right. Maps can be valuable tools not only for clarifying what food sources and/or land availability already exists in an area (in the shape of farms, home growers, orchards, local food retail outlets, etc.) but also in helping a community to plan what more local food projects and sites are needed if it is to achieve its own food resilience. For these reasons, a number of Transition initiatives, including those in Brixton, Lewes and Dunbar, are exploring how food- or land-mapping projects could help them.

On a larger scale, the Transition Network has teamed up with mapping experts Geofutures and the editor of *The Land* magazine Simon Fairlie (author of the seminal 2008 article 'Can Britain Feed Itself?'

described in the Introduction[4]) to devise a web-based project that will show how much land is needed to feed communities around the UK. In short, it will show the food footprints of communities on an interactive map, so that they can then plan their local food networks accordingly. Maps already created by Geofutures (such as that featured on page 168) show that the footprints of larger communities overlap and swallow up land occupied by neighbouring villages, towns and cities – obviously having large food-access implications for the swallowing and the swallowed. It is hoped that this project will be a valuable resource for Transition initiatives and other community groups planning how to keep themselves fed in uncertain times. See Mark Thurstain-Goodwin's article, below, for a more detailed account of the project.

As part of the Making Local Food Work programme, the Campaign to Protect Rural England (CPRE), working with Sustain, has funding to roll out a local food mapping project across the UK. At the time of writing it is running pilot projects in Hastings, Kenilworth, Knutsford, Leicester, Sheffield and Totnes,

The map of food
Mark Thurstain-Goodwin

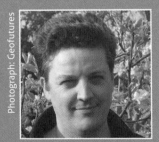

Photograph: Geofutures

As Transition communities start considering how they will feed themselves in a post-oil economy, they immediately face a major challenge in finding, combining and understanding all the data they need to help them plan a resilient food supply. One Transition project getting underway will use geographic information science (GIS) provided by our company Geofutures to create a food-mapping model for Totnes. The Network hopes that this model will then be refined and made available online.

GIS enables us to process huge volumes of data and tie each data point to a location on a digital map. The technology therefore allows us to perceive patterns and variations instantly, and to bring together multiple data sets for a location, helping us understand their combined effects. Most importantly, maps are easy to use – especially now that fast web access makes them available on any browser. You don't need to be an expert to understand peaks and troughs, highs and lows, and see immediately how your own community fits into the data landscape.

This project builds on Simon Fairlie's work that estimates how much land is needed to produce food, fuel and fibre per head of the population, together with the approximate share of production within concentric food zones serving a community [based on Growing Communities' zones diagram, shown on page 16]. We define the productive zone around a community, based on these combined approaches, as a 'foodshed'.

As a pilot, we'll build a GIS model combining demand-side data for Totnes – the size of the population and its food needs – with all the different factors affecting potential supply, such as land availability, current land use including gardens and woodlands, topography, soil types and so on. Mapping this combined picture makes it far easier to understand the size of the foodshed and how far each food zone needs to extend to feed the population.

The ultimate aim is to optimise food production between communities, recognising that different environments suit different types of production and that all foodsheds will have to be interconnected. While relocalising our economies is vital, we also need to recognise that it will be a rare community that can source all its needs locally.

Vegetable production, at the garden, nursery or field scale, is most likely to be able to meet local needs, but we also need protein, traditionally from meat and dairy, and carbohydrates, commonly from cereals and potatoes. If we recognise that some production will have to take place away from the immediate area of a community to be efficient, especially to meet the needs of our major conurbations, we need a combined picture for the whole country to allow us to optimise our planning now.

Based on simple online maps and IT infrastructure developed by Geofutures, users will eventually be able to view and add to local-scale current land-use data, and add ideas, production estimates, data and assumptions. Once the model has been tested further and refined with this information, it should be available to use as a hands-on planning tool on the web for any community to use. That's the bit I find most exciting. The technology is great but it's nothing without the data. Here's an opportunity for GIS mapping to be used for something incredibly important, bringing potential benefits to every community. At the same time, these communities will also play a vital part in collecting the information we need to build up as accurate and useful a picture as possible.

Mark Thurstain-Goodwin is the founder and Managing Director of Geofutures, and an active member of Transition City Bath. The paper produced by Geofutures and Transition Town Totnes, Can Totnes and District Feed Itself?, *is available at http://tinyurl.com/nkq7h8.*

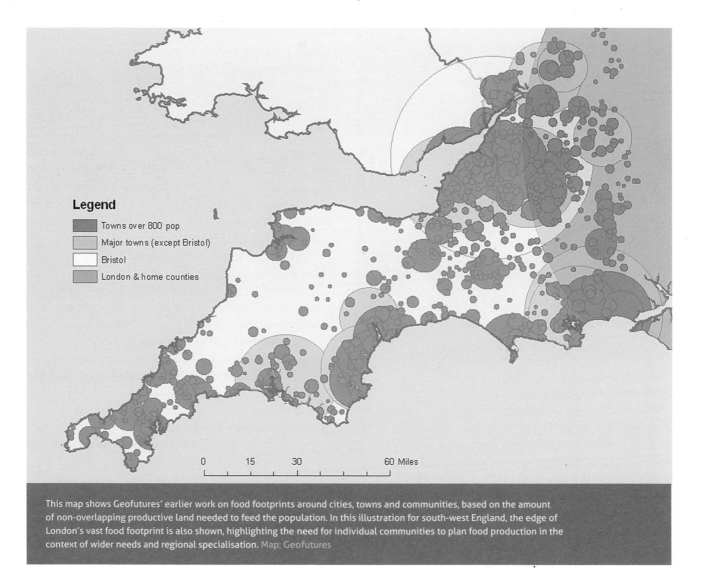

This map shows Geofutures' earlier work on food footprints around cities, towns and communities, based on the amount of non-overlapping productive land needed to feed the population. In this illustration for south-west England, the edge of London's vast food footprint is also shown, highlighting the need for individual communities to plan food production in the context of wider needs and regional specialisation. Map: Geofutures

where local volunteers are undertaking research on their local food networks (including interviewing consumers, producers, retailers and restaurant owners). Data will then be collated and made available for public use. In Totnes, the project is being conducted with the support and cooperation of Transition Town Totnes, and is building on the research already undertaken by the local food guide team. The hope is that both the research process and the presentation of the evidence will help local residents to source local food more easily, connect with others on the food supply chain, and help to shape the local food network in their area. This is of course an ideal project for UK-based Transition initiative participants to become involved in, and the Transition Network is in discussion with CPRE over how the project can be extended across other Transition groups nationwide. But that is not to say that mapping projects cannot also happen independently, and if CPRE's work is not coming to a town near you, don't let that be a reason not to get mapping yourselves.

Resources

See page 196 for Food and land mapping and page 203 for Local food – general.

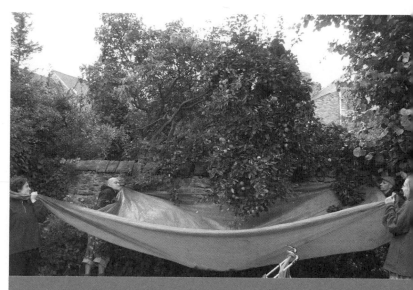

Abundance volunteers collecting the fruits of their labours.
Photograph: Anne-Marie Culhane

Glut and gleaning projects

One of the activities carried out by Transition City Nelson's Open Orchard Project (see page 97) is to harvest fruit from trees around the city, but for some other food projects the gleaning of community gluts can be and is their central focus. For example, the food growing cooperative Organic Lea in London's Waltham Forest has run its own Scrumping Project for a few years – tracking down, mapping and harvesting fruit trees across the borough.

Another similar project is scouring the branches of fruit trees further north, in the city of Sheffield. There, the arts-based community food initiative Grow Sheffield has created the Abundance project (not to be confused with the ABUNDANCE project, based in Brixton, see page 87), an urban fruit-harvesting initiative that scouts for fruit trees and willing volunteer pickers across the city. Since 2007 the project's

organisers Anne-Marie Culhane and Stephen Watts have seen it expand rapidly, harvesting eighty trees in its first season and 200 in 2008. It has also grown from one to two groups of harvesters, and up to 300 volunteers in total. At the peak of 2008's gleaning frenzy, teams were collecting a tonne of local fruit a week, which they then distributed among local organisations such as homeless shelters, health schemes and community cafes. The 40 per cent of harvested fruit that wasn't good enough for distributing in this way was pressed and juiced. As part of the Abundance project, volunteers have helped to track down and map local fruit trees, and the organisers have also run pruning workshops to encourage year-round care of the trees. Inspired by the glut-and-gleaning work going on in Sheffield, a sister organisation has now emerged – Abundance Manchester – that is doing similar work in its own urban territory. For more information and tips based on the Abundance experience, download a free copy of the group's handbook from its website, www.growsheffield.com.

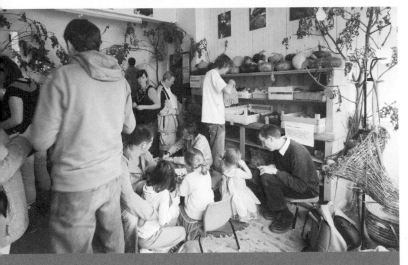

Members of the Sheffield community at Encounter Abundance – the free fruit-exchange shop project run by the group.
Photograph: Peter Hodge

Projects such as these help to galvanize community respect and care for the edible trees in the community's midst, transforming residents' relationship to their place of home, its trees and each other. There are of course other kinds of gluts that community projects could choose to focus their energies on, and activities might include organising stalls, swaps (see page 173), collections or cook-ups of home- or community-grown produce. These are all fun, sociable, delicious events that help to make sure all food grown in the community is eaten up and enjoyed.

Resources
See page 201 for Glut and gleaning.

Linking with local currencies

At the time of writing, the Transition initiatives of Totnes and Lewes in the UK are the only two to have initiated their own local currencies – the Totnes and Lewes pounds. They currently both operate with 1 pound notes, but in Lewes new denominations of 5, 10 and 21 Lewes pound notes are to be launched. As the Transition Network grows, more initiatives, including those in Brixton, Stroud and Southampton, may well follow in Totnes's and Lewes's footsteps, creating their own local currencies that will circulate within their community and help to strengthen and plough profit back into the local economy. A local currency is therefore a natural companion to any local food network, and as its circulation spreads it can encourage local trade through all the money-based stages of the food supply chain.

Local currency work in Lewes and Totnes is in its early stages, but both have managed to link the pound projects to their local food network in some way. In Totnes, the local food guide is sold in Totnes pounds, and its use is encouraged at all Transition events where money changes hands. In Lewes, the local Harveys brewery produced a special beer, 'Quids in' to commemorate the pound's launch, and contributed a 'Quids in' hamper to the prize lottery run through the individual numbers printed on each pound note. In both towns, the local pound is taken and actively supported by numerous food retailers, some of whom pay their local suppliers with it or who offer special deals for customers using the currencies. As the local food networks grow, scope for local currencies will grow with it. One day, farmers' markets or food co-ops could be run almost entirely on local currencies, and it may even become frowned upon to try to purchase local products with currencies issued by national, stock-exchange-weathered banks.

Resources
See page 202 for Linking with local currencies.

Local food challenges

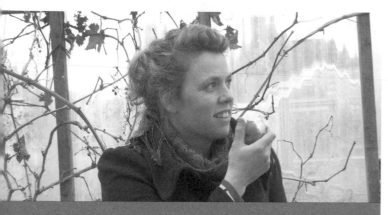

Beth Tilston from Eat The Change tucking into a local apple.
Photograph: Beth Tilston

In 2005, Vancouver residents James MacKinnon and Alissa Smith came up with the idea of challenging themselves to eat only produce sourced within a 100-mile radius of their home, for twelve months. They documented their experiences on the web (www.100milediet.org), and their idea soon grabbed much media attention and popularity among local food supporters worldwide. There has since been a flurry of publicly and privately conducted variations on the local-food-challenge theme. One of the better-known examples of this was undertaken by the American author Barbara Kingsolver and her family, eloquently and movingly described in her book *Animal, Vegetable, Miracle*.

Back in the UK, the Eat The Change initiative ran its pilot project for one week in September 2008, when 119 people in Bristol, Brighton, London and beyond agreed to "eat entirely local, organic, wild and plastic-free food or solely local or organic, wild or a combination of such foods for a whole week . . ."[5] On the back of the pilot's success, the project is being rolled out with an even larger following in 2009. Spearheading the initiative is Fergus Drennan (who set out to eat only foraged food for one year – see his article on wild food foraging on page 40), Beth Tilston (eating only food sourced within a 100-mile radius of her home) and Mark Boyle (who is living for a year without using oil at all – which includes eating only organic, non-packaged food).

Another UK-based example of a local food challenge comes from the Scottish region of Fife, where hundreds of residents chose to eat a Fife diet between October 2007 and October 2008 under the gaze of much media attention, and to the acclaim of other local food supporters nationwide.

One of the main benefits of embarking on a food challenge of this kind is to promote local food and encourage access to it. But it is much more than an awareness-raising exercise. As Beth Tilston (also a member of Transition City Brighton and Hove) points out, eating within a 100-mile radius has led her to discover a reconnection with the people and the places that produce her food, an interest in the stories attached to it, and an appreciation of her own cultural identity. The challenge has also allowed participants to boost their health, cut down on their own energy footprints, highlight the failings within their local food networks, compare local food accessibility in different parts of the country, and (it is hoped) prove that it is possible to eat well on a 'locavore' diet.

Fife's local food challenge provides a good example of community benefits that can arise from such a project, as Fife-diet participants are now pulling together to form a food co-op to support their local food network. Anyone thinking about embarking on such a challenge might bear in mind that the findings of local-food-challenge participants could be of great value to their local Transition or other community food groups. These groups could in turn help to promote and share the food-challenge experiences with the community at large.

Resources

See page 202 for Local food challenges.

Producer collaboration

'Producer collaboration' is a vague term to cover all the different projects, ideas and plans that could arise from greater community interaction with local producers – something that, at the time of writing, is being pursued by the food group of Transition Town Totnes (see Teresa Anderson's article on page 181). Many of the projects already featured in this book do of course encourage and facilitate more consumer–producer interaction and shortening of food supply chains, but it may well prove beneficial to try to build these relationships as a project focus in itself.

Forging these links can take years, not least because many farmers and growers have little time to spare out of their working hours. But if it is made clear that it will be to their benefit to interact with their consumers and that this can help them to establish a larger, more secure market for their goods, they may well feel encouraged to participate. Open Space days, community–farmer workshops, or even picnics and fairs might be ways of bridging the divide that has recently swallowed up these precious community interactions.

Community groups wanting to link in with local producers in this way could hunt them down by contacting the Soil Association, looking through local food directories or getting in touch with existing farmer co-ops or producer groups in the area. The Soil Association has in fact expressed a keen willingness to support and help facilitate producer–community interaction through its discussions with the Transition Network, and this opens up many exciting possibilities for Transition groups wanting to make these links. A wide range of inspired ideas and projects may emerge from creating space for these relationships to develop, as would an appreciation of the needs, hopes and aims of the respective other parties. And it would certainly serve to strengthen the local food network as a whole.

Resources

See page 206 for Producer collaboration.

Research

Undertaking background research will often be a part of the set-up of any local food project (see Step 2 on page 176), but carrying out research projects at the outset, before solid ideas have formed, can also point community groups towards plans and in directions that may not otherwise have come to light. Undertaking research can, for example, help to gauge public opinion on local food issues, provide clear data on a community's local food network as it is, or establish what new food projects need to be initiated. The research process can be a community bonding exercise in itself, through involving door-to-door surveys, holding community meetings and interviewing people involved in the local food network.

Transition Town Brampton has placed a large emphasis on research to assess the lie of the land in order to help the group decide how to take local food work forward. This has included conducting a survey on local food issues among households in the community, commissioning a local graduate to draw up a 'Feed Brampton' report, and raising funds to pay consultants from Growing Well, a Cumbrian-based, organic-food-growing, social enterprise, to conduct a feasibility study into the potential setting-up of a community garden. Whether such work is taken on by local volunteers or by paid experts in the field, and whether or not they paint a positive picture of the situation or unearth myriad 'opportunities' for change, it will all be useful grist for the community mill.

Resources
See page 206 for Research.

Seed, plant and food swaps

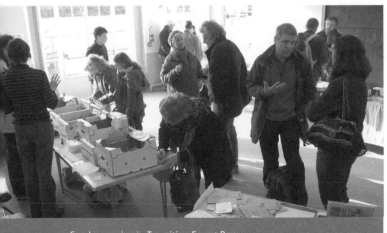

Seed swapping in Transition Forest Row.
Photograph: Transition Forest Row

Swapping events are a relatively simply and effective way of bypassing the small matter of money and focusing on the inherent value of the produce being exchanged. Seed swaps are particularly popular events within Transition initiatives and have featured on the listings of various groups, including those in Forest Row, Falmouth, Bristol and many other places besides. These seed-focused events are important for helping to preserve the genetic material of plants that has been largely hijacked by commercial, profit-driven seed companies, as well as protecting the important diversity of local and heritage varieties. They can piggyback on other community events, or constitute a day's outing in themselves – some of the larger events including local food cafes and talks and workshops alongside the actual swap. More formal seed-swapping events often ask for seed donations to be given to the organisers beforehand, so that they can be bagged, labelled and arranged on stalls. People attending the event then bring along more of their own seeds to swap. At less-structured swaps it is, of course, entirely up to the participants as to how produce is swapped and, for instance, how many home-grown cucumbers might be exchanged for a jar of blackcurrant jam. The money-free aspect of these swaps often makes for popular attendance as they are a refreshing change from the 'Spend, spend!' drama of the average high street.

Resources
See page 207 for Seed, plant and food swaps.

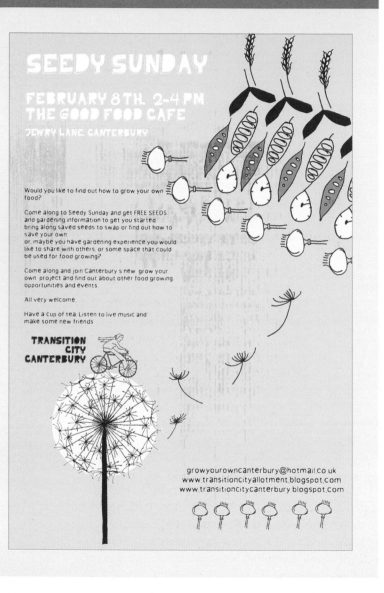

And more ideas still

- Community cafes or restaurants.
- Local food calendars.
- Jam, juice, wine, sauerkraut, seaweed, nettle or potato festivals!
- Local community pot-luck meals.
- Surprise farmer- and grower-appreciation parties.
- Recipe competitions and local recipe cookbooks.
- And all the many fabulous ideas you are yet to grow!

Chapter 16

THE LOCAL FOOD PROJECT AND BEYOND

If your bursting enthusiasm for local food hasn't already convinced you to put down this book and start gathering support for your new edible inspiration, then you may find the following of use on your community-food-project path. Below are suggested steps for setting up such a project, and ways of sharing and linking it to others within your community and beyond.

Steps to creating a community food project

These steps are suggestions for going about creating a community project around local food. Use them as guidelines and in the order that best suits your group (once you have one) and its needs. Some projects, for example, may already have an aim or even a site for their work before a group has formed around the idea (in which case you can dispense with Step 3), while others may start with an individual who simply has a clear desire to do something to strengthen local food in his or her area (in which case it may be helpful to start from Step 1 and work onwards). There will be other projects that are so small in scale that they do not necessitate all of the steps or taking on any structure or formality at all. If there is not yet an established Transition initiative in your community and you choose to focus your energies into getting it

going, or if you would like to set up a food group within an existing Transition initiative, then please refer to *The Transition Handbook* or the *Transition Primer* (freed to download at www.transitionnetwork.org) for steps and tips on how to go about it. For those who are still keen to set up a specific food project, whether in the context of a Transition group or not, then please read on.

1. Form a group

There are a number of ways you can drum up the company you need for forming a group and starting a community project. Begin by looking in all the likely places for fellow or potential local food supporters – a local Transition initiative, its food group, other food-focused groups, environmental groups, food co-ops and box schemes. You could put a call for group members out on their mailing lists, chat to others at their meetings or events, put an ad in their newsletters or magazines, or pin up posters on community noticeboards in your area. If you already have a clear idea about what kind of project you'd like to get stuck into, and what skills you need to make it happen, you can of course be more specific about who you direct your ads and call-outs to. For example, if you know you need someone experienced in growing food, you could hunt for them among local gardening or allotment groups. If you don't yet have a clear project plan, then existing food groups are the perfect places to explore ideas. But if you do open your ideas up to the wider community in this way, be prepared to involve and include everyone that comes along, and to make the most of the skills that they bring to the group. Asking new members to be clear about what skills they already have from the outset is important for the group to be able to plan and assign roles accordingly.

2. Find out what's out there and forge links

If you haven't already built up a good understanding of existing food-focused groups and initiatives while seeking fellow cohorts, this is an important step in seeing how your project will fit into the existing local food network – or indeed, in identifying exactly what types of project are needed in your area. Through networking you can develop contacts that may be an important source of support, sharing and inspiration once your project is fully fledged and kicking. And, when you are further down the line, you can make your presence and aims known to others through articles in local papers, giving presentations and attending food-related events in the community. Other than those groups mentioned in Step 1, you can build up an idea of what is happening in your area through looking in local food guides, doing web searches, and chatting with people who run health-food shops, farms and other food schemes. Of course, if there is an existing food group in your area it may well already have all the contacts you could wish for. Have a look at page 180 for a more in-depth discussion of how to build up a local food network beyond and around your project, and how a food group can play an important role in making this happen.

3. Identify what type of project you want to work on

This book covers a number of different types of food project to get you thinking about what you could take on yourselves. Here are some tips and questions you might want to ask yourselves during that process.

- Why do you want to set up a community food project? Give each group member the opportunity to express why he or she wants to be part of such a project and what he or she hopes to get out of it. This might give a clearer idea of the direction you all hope to go in.

- What areas of local food interest you? This is an obvious question but one that it can be easy to overlook in a group context. Again, giving each group member the chance to explore where his or her own local food passions lie might suggest a project shape and idea.

- How much spare time do you have between you to dedicate to the project?

- How many of you are there? An easy enough question to answer, but try to take on something that is appropriate to the amount of shared work you can all handle. All the projects described in this book list the number of participants involved – use this as an indication of the kind of person-power needed for a similar project of that size.

- Do you want to do a one-off project, or are you prepared to take on one that requires long-term commitment?

- What knowledge and resources do you already have between you, i.e. land, skills, tools, gardening experience, etc.? List all of these during a group brainstorming session and see if there is an obvious food project to match them with.

- What local food projects are needed in your area? If you haven't already covered this in Step 2, you can do it now. Research what's out there and determine what gaps need filling.

- Do you have any access to funds? If you have funds from the outset (from other group funds, personal savings or other means), then you may want to shape the project in accordance with how much you already have to spend. Having no funds at all is by no means a reason not to go ahead – many of the projects in this book were built up on little or no financial input, or with the help of grants, loans or donations that were pulled in along with way. In the UK we are fortunate to have a number of funders keen to support local food initiatives – there is money there for the taking (see Funding, grants and loans, page 197, in the Resources section).

4. Conjure up positive visions

As noted in Chapter 1, visioning is an integral part of the Transition process that can be usefully applied to the set-up of any community food project, helping to define the group's hopes and goals for the path it is about to embark on. For more about visioning see page 30.

5. Get planning

At this point, it might be a good idea to do the following.

- Identify a list of agreed principles to guide the project – including how, as a group, you define healthy, local food and sustainable food production. Many of the projects in this book and across the local food movement have varied definitions, so it is important that you clarify what boundaries you are and aren't prepared to cross. These can be amended and referred to over time, when necessary.

- Consider your group's structure. How will decisions be made? What roles and tasks are members to take on? See 'Organisations giving financial, legal or organisational advice' on page 205 of the Resources section for sources of advice on formal organisational structure, or refer to the *Transition Primer* (available as a free download at www.transitionnetwork.org) for more information on the Transition model.

- How will you source all the tools, land, voluntary assistance, etc. that you need to get the project going? Plan and draw up a timetable you hope to work to.

- Will you be going for organic certification? If so, you can seek assistance from the Soil Association, the Wholesome Food Association or other accreditation bodies (details of both are given under 'Local food – general' in the Resources section). If you choose to be accredited by the Soil Association, it may well be worth pooling the costs and going for its group certification scheme between a group of growers, sellers, etc.

- Are there legal regulations that relate to your project? Make sure you are aware of all the relevant health, food safety, planning and trading standards from the outset. There are organisations and governmental bodies that will be able to advise you – see 'Organisations giving financial, legal or organisational advice' on page 205 of the Resources section.

6. Enlist help

A good way of firmly embedding a local food project within a community is by giving other community members the chance to contribute in some way. As mentioned in the 'sowing and reaping' theme in Chapter 1 (see page 30), asking for help within the community can have surprisingly pleasing results. You may even find that people are willing to offer their professional services (such as marketing, web design, bookkeeping and legal work) at reduced rates if they are supportive of your aims. Lastly, make good use of the many local, regional and national organisations that are doing work around local food. They are very experienced in the field and many of them can offer helpful advice and support, and direct you to sources of funding. The most prominent ones are listed under 'Organisations giving financial, legal or organisational advice' (page 205) in the Resources section, but there may well be other, smaller ones in your area that you can turn to.

7. Honour the elders

This is particularly relevant in the context of the local food project. As we move down the slope away from a peak in oil production, the elder folk in our communities will be a valuable source of ideas, skills and knowledge on how to feed our families without the help of cheap energy. The farming community is a good place to look for this expertise, not least because the average UK farmer is approaching retirement age. Those that are older still can provide a direct window to a past, less frivolous time. How did they run their farms before cheap oil was readily available? What tools, animal power and fertilisers did they use? Who did they sell their produce to and how was it transported? Even if your project is not agricultural in nature, there are also many elder people among the non-farming communities for whom growing their own food was once a necessity and a way of life – and they may be able to advise, inspire new directions or participate in your work. After all, one of guerrilla gardener Richard Reynolds' most supportive and active 'troops' is his own 93-year-old grandmother (known for guerrilla purposes as Margot 623), proving that it is never too late to get earth under the fingernails. Bringing the elder community members into your work helps to reconnect the project and other project members with local, social history and the place where you live, as well as helping to encourage community inclusivity and a good mix of ages within your group.

8. Let it go where it wants to go

Resist the urge to be rigid about your intentions for the food project at the expense of implementing necessary changes or letting others have a say. The obvious word to use in this context is of course 'organic' – allow your project to grow with the energy of the group and the community assistance, passion and input that nourishes it; unpolluted by attempts to restrain it, control its context or turn it into something it is not.

9. Make your project known

Publicise your efforts and make others in your community take notice of what you're up to. This is an important way of making your work go further and of allowing local food thinking to reach a wider audience – so it might be a good plan to build in time for self-promotion from the beginning. There may well be incredible people in your midst whose brilliance is just waiting to be triggered and inspired by someone else's dynamism, so be bold. (See the

'Enable sharing and networking' principle on page 32 for more ideas.)

10. Harvest your data as well as your food

The more data that is collected by home growers and local food producers on the ground, the more hard evidence we have of the benefits of this kind of food production – and the more ammunition we will have to help persuade those with a preference for numbers and figures that local, small-scale growing is indeed a financially viable and all-round sensible thing to do. Whether you are growing food in your own garden, running a food co-op or setting up a community forest garden, collecting figures on how much you grow and trade can be an invaluable source of information for your local food network and the wider movement. This kind of data can also be of great value when applying for funding or in promoting your project. Harvesting the figures may simply involve having a pair of scales and an exercise book and getting into the habit of weighing and recording everything as you pick it. It could then be the role of the local food group to collate this information for public use.

11. Look, think and act beyond your project

Read on for ideas and tips on how to expand, link and share the scope of your work.

Beyond the local food project

Up to this point our focus has been mainly on the individual food project itself and how it runs and evolves. But now we will shift the focus outwards, to see how the project could help others, and also what work is needed beyond the food project – both within a community and on a local food movement-wide basis.

Sharing project experiences

The Growing Communities food initiative described on pages 158-63 provides a good example of how, once a project has found its feet and established its financial independence, it can begin to move beyond its own walls and look at how its experiences, knowledge, skills and lessons learned might be of help to others at the start of their food-project journey. If project members

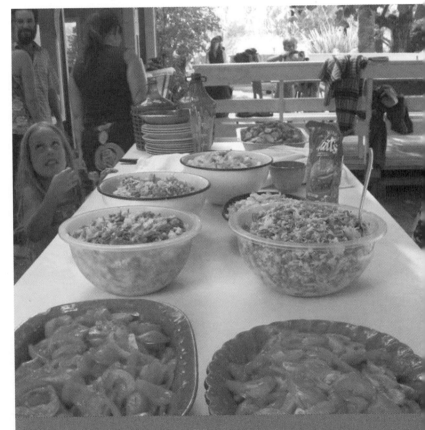

A meal from the fields in El Manzano, Chile.
Photograph: Ecoescuela El Manzano

have the time and energy to be able to embark on this kind of sharing exercise, their assistance will most likely be of huge benefit to other budding local foodies, and can help to further the aims of the local food movement at large. Ways of doing this include running open days, holding training workshops or courses, offering apprenticeships, giving talks, producing manuals or making your set-up materials publicly available on the Internet or by post. You may even find extra hands to help in the running of your own project in the process, or new directions and ideas may present themselves as you let new people in.

The food group: linking projects and building a local food network

As we have mentioned elsewhere, a food project's reach of influence will be significantly multiplied if it embeds itself within a network of relationships – with other relevant initiatives, schools, local government, environmental action groups and the like. And one of the most effective ways of facilitating open sharing and communication throughout this growing network is by having a group or hub in place to support, inspire, focus and connect local food work in your area – a group that will take on a similar holding role to that of the Transition Network (though on a much smaller scale). Such is one of the main functions of a Transition food group, or an organisation such as Grow Sheffield. If you are considering setting up a group of this kind, do try to avoid wasting precious time trying to replicate what already exists. If there are already effective local food groups or organisations in your community, it is worth linking in with them instead. In the beginning, the group is likely to be dependent upon volunteers. But over time it may become more sophisticated, and could take on more formal tasks and roles. Food-group members may, for example, choose to:

- take on an intermediary and connecting role between farmers and consumers, helping to communicate the community's needs to the farmers and vice versa (as the Transition Town Totnes's food group is setting out to do – see page 134)

- help to set up and oversee the sharing of tools, kitchens and processing facilities for local producers

- hold a database or directory of all local farmers, producers and home growers to facilitate networking and sharing between them

- hold regular Open Space events or public consultation sessions to assess the changing needs of the community, the farmers and growers

- build up a seed bank of local, heritage varieties that local growers can use and replenish each year

- provide advice and funding ideas for fledgling projects

- build up an accurate map of local food activity in the area and have a clear idea of what new work might be needed, so as to steer new local food entrepreneurs in directions most appropriate for their community

- work on developing the food section of the community's Energy Descent Action Plan (EDAP).[1] The food group should be well placed and well connected to take on this task, visioning the local food network of the future and casting back to the present to come up with a plan of action. Once this part of the EDAP is in place, it will be a useful 'map' that can help guide and realise local food activity in the community

- collect and collate information on yields and growing methods based on the data shared by local growers, farmers and food projects.

The latter idea leads to an important point – that there needs to be careful planning within communities to ensure that the majority of our food needs can be met locally, and that there isn't, for example, an over-abundance of cheese produced in one community and excessive amounts of apples grown in another. A food group will ideally have a bird's eye view, an active appreciation of the benefits of polycultural growing and the necessary contacts to ensure this doesn't happen. Mapping and directory projects can be of useful assistance along the way, as can support from the Transition Network and other supportive organisations in the local food movement.

The Transition Town Totnes food group

Teresa Anderson

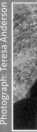

Photograph: Teresa Anderson

Food is so visceral. Everybody understands its importance. The growing and marketing of food has become a potent symbol for all that is good and bad about the economics, politics, community and health of the world today. Food becomes a practical means through which we can channel our convictions. The solutions are both immediate (start digging!) and long-term (strengthening farmers' links to local markets), and can involve small or large steps. But however you go about being part of a shift towards local food, it is invariably an empowering experience – you can start growing vegetables tomorrow and know that you are already contributing to your own resilience and security. Perhaps for all of these reasons, the food group is one of the busiest and most participatory of those that make up Transition Town Totnes (TTT).

In TTT's first year, the food group focused on projects that encouraged community involvement, which would make our presence felt. The work was visible within the town itself, such as nut trees in public spaces and local food guides in the shops. We welcome anyone bringing ideas and energy to the food group, and there has been a steady flow of new ideas and people to keep us busy.

Now that the group has laid down substantial roots in the community, we are starting to branch out and look further afield. The next step is about supporting farmers to strengthen their links to local consumers, and to grow as much food as possible to meet local needs.

The food group has a special role to play in the Transition Town. Like a good family meal, there will always be something for everyone. It can sometimes be a little over-ambitious, but the group's work is always satisfying. The most important thing to remember, though, is that everyone feels welcome at the table.

Teresa Anderson is the coordinator of Transition Town Totnes's food group, and the information and advocacy officer for the Gaia Foundation (see www.totnes. transitionnetwork.org and www.gaiafoundation.org).

Bristol's food in transition

Claire Milne

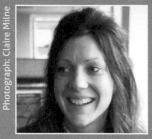

Photograph: Claire Milne

Boasting the first-ever edible chocolate bar and, of course, Bristol Cream sherry, Bristol itself historically imported most of its food in exchange for pins, guns, tweed, wool and, sadly, war. Bristol today, however, is blessed with an abundance of amazing urban food initiatives working hard to reconnect people with where their food comes from and helping to create Carolyn Steel's vision of Sitopia (from the ancient Greek *sitos*, food, and *topos*, place). As well as Bristol's myriad community-food projects, hundreds of fruit and nut trees were planted across Bristol in 2008 as part of Transition Bristol's virtual orchard. By buying trees in bulk we were able to sell them online at wholesale prices and teach people how to care for their tree when they came to collect it.

Transition Bristol is now working with other city-wide organisations to develop a sustainable food strategy for Bristol – which will form the basis of the food strand of our EDAP. We plan to start by exploring our existing food chain – identifying where Bristol's food currently comes from, how it's distributed and how much land is needed to feed Bristol's population – now and in the future. We'll then focus on mapping our food chain and identifying alternative models based on local and sustainable food production, sustainable transport links and, most importantly, on forging connections that nourish both people and the environment. A local project, Eat Somerset, has been working with local producers and local retailers to explore the barriers to getting more local food into Bristol, and slowly but surely relationships between local farmers and Bristol communities are being rebuilt.

We are also working with Bristol Food Hub to explore how to move beyond mobilising the 'usual suspects' – inspiring diverse communities to transform their relationships with food. Our seasonal food celebrations Berries 'n' Beans and Share the Harvest have started this process: using a positive celebratory approach to food, rather than a preachy one that tends to engage only the low-hanging fruit, so to speak.

Our Eat the Change campaign at harvest time in 2008 inspired hundreds of people across Bristol and around the country to try to eat only local, organic food, free from plastic packaging, for one week. Important learnings were enjoyed, revealing just how challenging something so natural and simple has become.

So what does the future hold for food in Bristol? First and foremost we need to wean ourselves off our addictions to foods that are not just crippling our health but are also hampering nature's ability to sustain us. Rather more excitingly, we need to start rebuilding relationships between communities, local farmers and other food producers so that everyone starts to play a more active role in the food we eat – and awakens to the realisation that our relationships with food can transform our lives in a profound way.

Claire Milne is a consultant for Bristol City Council, working on resurrecting the local food network across the city. She is also an active participant in Transition City Bristol food projects, is coordinator of the Bristol Food Hub and is developing the Transition Network's food and farming strategy discussed opposite (see www. transitionbristol.net, www.bristolfoodhub.org).

The scale and nature of a food group's work may vary depending on the community context it is part of. The two articles on the preceding pages describe the local food activities of Transition initiatives in two contrasting settings – a rural market town and a city – Totnes and Bristol. Together they give an idea of the kind of work that is carried out in coordinating or linking up local food activity at either end of the rural-to-urban spectrum.

Local food across the Transition Network

On an even larger scale, there is much sharing that can occur, and work to be done, at the level of the Transition Network. It is the Network's role to support the various communities embarking on Transition and, with regard to food, to empower them to create and strengthen their own local food networks. To enable this work, Transition Bristol's Claire Milne (see her article on local food in her city, opposite) is drawing up Transition Network's Food Strategy, which will pull together the knowledge and resources necessary to allow many more community food projects, similar to those detailed in this book, to flourish. Once the Strategy has been rolled out the Network will be able to support groups in the food-focused directions they choose to take – whether, for example, it is in developing the food section of their Energy Descent Action Plan, trying to establish relationships with local food producers in their area, or working to transform the food-procurement policies of local institutions.

Three strands of this Strategy have already been mentioned – work with the Soil Association to encourage producer–community collaboration, the mapping project with the Council for the Protection of Rural England, and Geofutures' food mapping initiative (see page 166 for both). Establishing working relationships with other local food organisations such as these is central to this Strategy and, besides those already noted, the Network has also forged links with Sustain, the Federation of City Farms and Community Gardens, the New Economics Foundation, the Permaculture Association, the Food Ethics Council and Garden Organic (see pages 204, 192, 204, 210, 210 and 200 respectively for contact details). Just as it is crucial for food projects across a community to work together, share their resources and open their doors to others building on similar aims, this also needs to happen at the strategic level if food relocalisation is going to be effective, inclusive and thorough on a wide scale.

One further and important strand of the Strategy's work that will facilitate greater sharing between community-based projects is the food web portal – an online site that will act as a directory and forum for food work across the Network and beyond. At the time of writing there is a team of dedicated Transitioners working on the pilot version of this portal and it is expected to develop into a key component of the Transition Network's online presence (keep an eye on www.transitionnetwork.org for more information). The food web portal will assemble, categorise and deliver food-project information from Transition groups around the world, building up a cyber-representation of the local food networks we are growing on the ground. This will be a crucial resource for everyone involved in localising food – not only for finding out what else is out there but also for assisting the flow of communication, knowledge, plans, photos and ideas between projects.

In the meantime, while the Strategy is being tied together and its various projects are being created, anyone interested in contributing suggestions to the Network's food work can do so by responding to the 'Transitioning our food – strategy & ideas' subject posted on the Transition food forum (see www.transitiontowns.org/forum/forum.php?id=12). Your input is welcome!

Some closing thoughts

We hope you have found this book useful and informative, and that you now feel inspired to create or be involved in a local food project within your community, and to be a part of the local food networks that are rapidly appearing around the globe. Your timing is good. Our cultural focus is shifting from the outward-looking exploration of the new, the far away, the complex and the illusory to a reconnection with what's familiar, local, simple and real. As the castles of the global economy are being swallowed up by the sands they were built upon, communities from rural Devon to urban New Zealand are coming to re-evaluate the quality of the soil beneath their feet and feel how its health nourishes their own. And as our taste for cheap energy and cultural excess melts our ice caps, poisons our wildlife and dries up our oilfields, we are realising the necessity of living with care and light-footed intelligence. By collectively demystifying the contents of the global pantry and by sourcing, growing and producing food independently of centralised, fragile and detrimental food trades, we are rediscovering our own worth as community members – people capable of interacting with and shaping the food landscapes around us. We are bringing our food culture home because we have to. And while we know we can't move mountains, we are remembering that we can plant seeds.

Photograph: istock photo

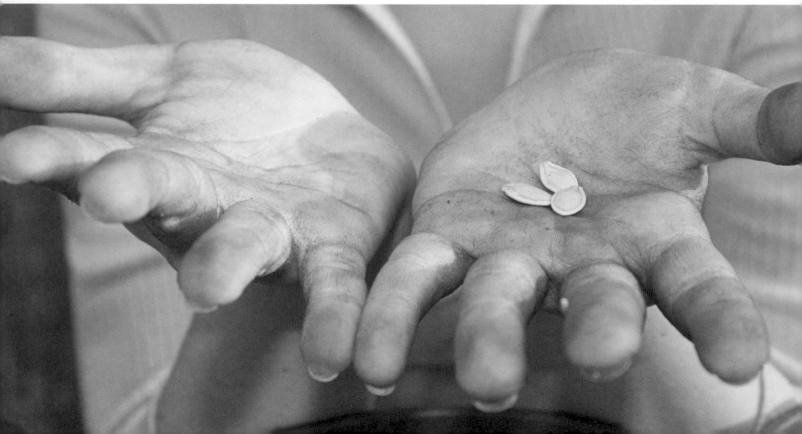

REFERENCES

Introduction

1 Cabinet Office (2008) *Food: An analysis of the issues.* Revision D, August 2008. The Strategy Unit. Available at www.cabinetoffice.gov.uk/media/cabinetoffice/strategy/assets/food/food_analysis.pdf.

2 Hansen, J., Sato, M., Kharecha, P., Beerling, D., Berner, R., Masson-Delmotte, V., Pagani, M., Raymo, M., Royer, D. L. and Zachos, J. C. (2008) 'Target Atmospheric CO_2: Where Should Humanity Aim?' *The Open Atmospheric Science Journal 2: 217-31.*

3 Thompson, S., Abdallah, S., Marks, N. & Simms, A. (2007) *The (un)happy planet index: An index of human well-being and environmental impact.* New Economics Foundation, London.

4 Mellanby, K. (1975) *Can Britain Feed Itself?* Merlin Press, London.

5 Fairlie, Simon (2007) 'Can Britain Feed Itself?', *The Land* 4, 18-25.

6 Owing to very high levels of grant applications, the National Lottery (which is overseeing the Local Food Fund) took the decision to suspend further acceptance of first-stage applicants in August 2009. See www.local-foodgrants.org for more information.

Chapter 1: The local food movement

1 Heinberg, Richard & Bomford, Michael (2009) *The Food and Farming Transition,* A report by the Post Carbon Institute, USA, available at www.postcarbon.org/food.

2 Jack Kloppenberg describes foodsheds as "self-reliant, locally or regionally based food systems comprised of diversified farms using sustainable practices to supply fresher, more nutritious foodstuffs to small-scale processors and consumers to whom producers are linked by the bonds of community as well as economy." Kloppenberg, J. (1991) 'Social theory and the de/reconstruction of agricultural science: a new agenda for rural sociology', *Sociologica Ruralis* 32(1): 519-48.

3 While the word 'community' can be used to refer to social groupings defined by, for example, interests, age, work or religion, in the context of this book it is used to describe those groupings that are linked to place, such as the community of people who share a village, town or city.

4 IGD (2009) *Shopper Trends 2009: Food shopping in a recession*, available at www.igd.com/index.asp?id=1&fid=2&sid=2&cid=629.

5 Mintel (2009) *Local Procurement Report*, available at http://oxygen.mintel.com/sinatra/reports/display/id=393577.

6 IGD (2005) *The local and regional food opportunity*, available at www.defra.gov.uk/foodrin/foodname/guides/pdf/localregfoodopps.pdf.

7 See Vandana Shiva's book *Soil Not Oil* (2008, Zed Books, London) for an eloquent justification of why strengthening local food networks in the developed world will also benefit farmers in poorer countries.

8 Soil Association (2008) *An inconvenient truth about food – neither secure nor resilient*, p.7. Available at www.soilassociation.org/web/sa/saweb.nsf/GetInvolved/food_security.html.

9 A study conducted in Cornwall by the New Economics Foundation found that a switch of just 1% of consumer spending away from supermarkets and towards local produce had the effect of increasing the income of local food businesses by a staggering £52 million each year, with all the jobs and economic security that came with it. New Economics Foundation (2002) *The Money Trail: Measuring your impact on the local economy using LM3*.

10 Assuming of course that they eat limited amounts of sustainably produced and sustainably sourced meat.

11 Organic growing is that done without the use of artificial chemical fertilisers, pesticides or the routine use of antibiotics and other drugs for livestock. According to Defra's definition of organic, however, up to seven identified pesticides are permitted as a last resort for growers and farmers of organic produce. The Soil Association permits only four (again, to be used as a last resort). For food to be sold as organic it has to be certified as such by the Soil Association or another organic certification body. See www.soilassociation.org.uk or www.defra.gov.uk for more information.

12 Biodynamic growing is an organic and holistic approach to food production gleaned from the anthroposophical work of Rudolf Steiner. It emphasises the interconnected relationships between plants, soil, the seasons and even the movement of the planets, and sees each biodynamic farm as a unique, living organism. See www.biodynamic.org.uk for more information.

13 Forest gardening, or agroforestry, works by mimicking and allowing for the natural growing patterns and relationships found in a forest. Pioneered by Robert Hart in Shropshire in the 1960s and for decades after, it is a highly productive system that requires minimal maintenance. See www.agroforestry.co.uk for more information.

14 Graham Bell, author of *The Permaculture Way*, offers the following helpful definition of permaculture: "Permaculture is the conscious design and maintenance of agriculturally productive systems which have the diversity, stability and resilience of natural ecosystems." However, permaculture is not just about agricultural productivity – it is a design principle that goes much further. David Holmgren, the co-founder (with Bill Mollison) of the concept, defines it thus: "Permaculture is a design system based on ecological principles which provides the organising framework for implementing a permanent or sustainable culture. It . . . draws together the diverse skills and ways of living which need to be rediscovered and developed to empower us to move from being dependent consumers to becoming responsible producers. In this sense, permaculture is not the landscape, or even the skills of organic gardening, sustainable farming, energy-efficient building or eco-village development as such, but can be used to design, establish, manage and improve these and all other efforts made by individuals, households and communities towards a sustainable future." (David Holmgren [2002], *Permaculture: Principles and Pathways Beyond Sustainability*. Holmgren Design Services.)

15 US activist Rebecca Solnit, *Hope in the Dark* (2004, Nation Books), quoted in Jess Worth, 'Power and Politics', *New Internationalist* 419, Jan/Feb 2009.

16 As described in the Transition Network's 'Who We Are and What We Do' document, available to download at www.transitionnetwork.org.

17 See Rob Hopkins' *The Transition Handbook* (2008, Green Books, Dartington) for more ideas of visioning exercises.

18 See *The Transition Handbook* for tips on writing press releases and making the most of public events.

19 We use the following definition of resilience, offered by Walker et al.: "Resilience is the capacity of a system to absorb disturbance and reorganise while undergoing change, so as to still retain essentially the same function,

structure, identity and feedbacks." Walker, B., Hollinger, C. S., Carpenter, S. R. & Kinzing, A. (2004) 'Resilience, adaptability and transformability in social-ecological systems', *Ecology and Society* 9(2): 5.

Chapter 3: Home garden growing in the community

1 Buncombe, Andrew (2006) 'The good life in Havana: Cuba's green revolution', *The Independent*, 8 August 2006.

2 Available at www.cosg.org.uk/greencuba.htm, on the website for the Cuban Organic Support Group.

3 Chamberlin, Shaun (2009) *The Transition Timeline*. Green Books, Dartington.

4 Horticultural Trades Association press release, 'HTA leaders have a positive outlook for the gardening industry', 25 September 2008, available at www.the-hta.org.uk/press_releases.asp.

5 Mesure, Susie (2008) 'The Good Life! Cooking and gardening with Jamie', *The Independent*, 16 March 2008.

6 Kelland, Kate (2008) 'More home grown veg as British, US belts tighten', available at http://in.reuters.com/article/worldNews/idININdia-33936720080606.

Chapter 4: Allotment provision and gardening for community groups

1 This calculation is based on figures taken from wartime allotments that produced on average □ tonne of food per plot. Stokes, G. W., pers. comm., National Society of Allotment and Leisure Gardeners, May 2009.

2 Available at www.allotment.org.uk./articles/Allotment-History.php.

3 University of Derby, Department of Communities and Local Government (2003) *Survey of Allotments, Community Gardens and City Farms*.

4 Vidal, John (2008) 'Coming up roses? Not any more as UK gardeners turn to vegetables', *The Guardian*, 22 March 2008.

5 A charity comprised of 3.6 million members that owns and runs historic properties and gardens around the UK. See www.nationaltrust.org.uk for more information.

6 It is estimated that the plots could yield around 2.6 million lettuces a year. They will be made available through the Landshare website (www.landshare.net).

7 Carlisle, D. (2003) 'Great oaks from little acorns grow', *Health Development Today* 4, 2003.

8 The Federation of City Farms and Community Gardens (2008) *The True Value of Community Farms and Gardens Research Report*.

9 LETS are community-based trading networks where members exchange goods and services, bypassing the need for money. See www.letslinkuk.net for more information.

Chapter 5: Garden shares

1 The following study is the most optimistic of those we've seen. Davies, Zoe G. et al., (2009) 'A national scale inventory of resource provision for biodiversity within domestic gardens', *Biological Conservation* 142(4): 761-71.

2 These figures are based on Simon Fairlie's calculations. See Fairlie, Simon (2007) 'Can Britain Feed Itself?', *The Land* 4, 18-25.

3 Shiva, Vandana (2008) *Soil Not Oil*. Zed Books, London, pp.115-18.

4 Open Space Technology is a powerful approach to running group meetings and discussions, commonly used by Transition groups and advocated in *The Transition Handbook*. It is largely unstructured and self-organising, so that participants determine what subjects are to be discussed around a central theme or question (such as

'How will Edinburgh feed itself beyond the age of cheap oil?'). They then plan the agenda for the event and partake in the small group discussions that interest them. See www.openspaceworld.org for more information.

Chapter 6: Community gardens

1 Community Land Trusts facilitate democratic, community ownership of land. See www.communitylandtrust.org.uk for case studies and advice on how to set up such trusts.

2 Quoted in David C. Taylor (2000) *Gerard Winstanley in Elmbridge*. Appleton Publications, Cobham.

3 Transcript of remarks by first lady Michelle Obama to US Department of Agriculture employees, 19 February 2009, available at www.usda.gov.

4 de Nies, Yunji (2009) 'Michelle Obama Breaks Ground', available at http://blogs.abcnews.com/politicalpunch/2009/03/michelle-obam-2.html.

5 Federation of City Farms and Community Gardens (FCFCG) in partnership with the Regeneration Exchange of the University of Northumbria (2008) *The True Value of Community Farms and Gardens.*

6 Gerard Winstanley (1649) *The True Leveller's Standard Advanced.*

7 See the following article for more information about this project: Catherine Sneed (2000) 'Seeds of Change', available at www.yesmagazine.org/article.asp?ID=381.

Chapter 7: Community orchards

1 Soil Association (2008) *An Inconvenient Truth About Food – Neither secure or resilient*, p.6. Available at www.soilassociation.org/web/sa/saweb.nsf/GetInvolved/food_security.html

2 Common Ground (1999) *Save Our Orchards* pamphlet.

3 Frank Hemming, Orchard Manager, Transition Town Hereford. Pers. comm., December 2008.

Chapter 8: Community supported agriculture

1 Harrison, M., Pilley, G. and Weir, N. (2008) *The Story of CSA in Stroud* (Appendices, section 11.1), available at www.stroudcommunityagriculture.org.

2 A meat-based diet is significantly more energy-intensive than one that is plant-based. Pimentel, David and Pimentel, Marcia (eds) (2008) *Food, Energy and Society* (3rd edn). CRC Press, Florida, pp.133-4.

Chapter 9: Farmers' markets

1 Pretty, Jules (2001) *Some Benefits and Drawbacks of Local Food Systems*. University of Essex.

2 United States Department of Agriculture (1996) *Farmers' Market Survey Report.*

Chapter 10: Food cooperatives

1 See www.cooperatives-uk.coop for more information on cooperatives in general.

2 Bath Farmers' Market, described on pages 115-17, has also experienced a rise in the popularity of its stalls despite the slowdown of the global economy.

Chapter 12: School projects on local food

1 *Sky News* 'Townie children think cows lay eggs', 28 February 2007, available at http://news.sky.com/skynews.

2 Local Authority Caterers Association (2004) School Meals Survey 2004. LACA, Woking.

Chapter 14: Expanding local food projects

1 Cardiff University (2003) *Relocalising the Food Chain: The role of creative public procurement*.

Chapter 15: Yet more inspired ideas

1 Defra (2008) *Waste Strategy Annual Progress Report 2007/08*, p.46, available at www.defra.gov.uk.

2 Brignall, Miles (2009) 'Last orders? Communities fight back', *The Guardian*, 21 March 2009.

3 Fearne, Andrew, et al. (2004) 'Measuring distributive and procedural justice in buyer/supplier relationships: an empirical study of UK supermarket supply chains', paper presented at the 88th Seminar of the European Association of Agricultural Economics, Paris, 2004, p.2.

4 Fairlie, Simon (2007) 'Can Britain Feed Itself?', *The Land* 4, 18-25.

5 See http://eatthechange.org/about/.

Chapter 16: The local food project and beyond

1 Drawing up an Energy Descent Action Plan (through open discussions and the compilation of an EDAP document) is central to the process of the Transition initiative, as a way of visioning and preparing for the years ahead. See Rob Hopkins' *The Transition Handbook* (2008, Green Books, Dartington).

RESOURCES

This section lists resources for local food community projects, many of which have been recommended by people on the ground. It isn't an exhaustive list of local food resources, but it is a starting point for the huge range that is out there. Contents are arranged alphabetically and correspond to the categories featured in the main part of this book, as well as including some other relevant subject areas. Each section is divided into books, organisations and websites. The projects described in detail in this book are listed here only if their contact details are on the web or are otherwise publicly available. All Transition initiatives cited in the book are listed in section 29, The Transition movement.

Contents

1	Allotments 190
2	Community composting 191
3	Community gardens 192
4	Community orchards 193
5	Community shops 193
6	Community Supported Agriculture schemes (CSAs) 193
7	Course centres 194
8	Expanding local food projects 195
9	Farmers' markets 195
10	Farming – general 195*
11	Food and land mapping 196
12	Food co-ops 197
13	Funding, grants and loans 197
14	Garden shares 199
15	General edible gardening 200
16	Glut and gleaning 201
17	The Great Reskilling 201
18	Home garden growing 202
19	Linking with local currencies 202
20	Local food challenges 202
21	Local food guides and directories 203
22	Local food events 203
23	Local food – general 203
24	Organisations giving financial, legal or organisational advice 205
25	Producer collaboration 206
26	Research 206
27	Seed, plant and food swaps 207
28	School projects on local food 207
29	The Transition movement 208
30	Yet more sources of help and interest 209

1 Allotments

Books

Clevely, Andi (2006) *The Allotment Book*. Collins.

Harrison, John (2009) *The Essential Allotment Guide*. Constable and Robinson.

Pears, Pauline (2007) *Successful Allotments: Green Essentials*. Impact Publishing.

Organisations and projects

The Awaiting Allotment Society
www.transitiontownwestkirby.org.uk/accesstoallotments.htm
Transition Town West Kirby's allotment project.

The National Society of Allotment and Leisure Gardeners (NSALG)
Corby, Northamptonshire
01536 266576
www.nsalg.org.uk

Organic Lea
London
www.organiclea.org.uk
020 8558 6880
A community allotment project that has grown into a flourishing cooperative, supplying its volunteers and other local residents with fresh organic food, running a local scrumping project and supplying stalls and a cafe. A report on the legality of selling allotment produce can be downloaded from the website.

St Ann's Allotments
Nottingham
0115 9110207
www.staa-allotments.org.uk

Websites

Allotment Growing
www.allotment.org.uk
An interesting and informative allotment blog complete with forums, tips and recipes.

www.allotmentssouthwest.org.uk
This non-profit-making organisation seeks to promote allotment gardening across the UK.

www.allotments-uk.com
All the information you might want to start up your own allotment project.

www.farmgarden.org.uk/ari
Run by the Federation of City Farms and Community Gardens – see section 3 (Community gardens) – the Allotments Regeneration Initiative has received lottery funding to run a network of mentors that can assist and advise communities wanting to set up allotment projects. Its website is very helpful – take a look at the factsheets in the resources section.

www.irishallotments.net
This website has a section on community groups and Transition Towns.

www.transitioncityallotment.blogspot.com
The blog site for the community allotment growers of Transition City Canterbury.

2 Community composting

Books

Appelhof, Mary and Fenton, Mary (1997) *Worms Eat My Garbage*. Flower Press.

Scott, Nicky (2006) *Composting: An easy household guide*. Green Books.

Organisations and projects

The Association for Organics Recycling (formerly The Composting Association)
Wellingborough, Northamptonshire
0870 160 3270
www.organics-recycling.org.uk

Community Composting Network (CCN)
Sheffield
0114 258 0483
www.communitycompost.org

Websites

www.growingwithcompost.org
This project provides training and support to community composting initiatives. Some of its resources are available online.

www.homecomposting.org.uk
A website run by Garden Organic with resources and advice for home composters, as well as how to get involved in the Master Composters scheme to promote composting in your local community.

www.wrap.org.uk/composting
Composting page from the Waste & Resources Action Programme.

3 Community gardens

Books

The Findhorn Community (2008) *The Findhorn Garden Story*. Findhorn Press.

Kirby, Ellen and Peters, Elizabeth (eds) (2008) *Community Gardening*. Brooklyn Botanic Garden.

Reynolds, Richard (2008) *On Guerrilla Gardening: A handbook for gardening without boundaries*. Bloomsbury.

Organisations and projects

BS3 Community Smallholding
www.transitionbs3.co.uk
Transition BS3's thriving food-growing project in Bristol.

Diggin' It Community Garden
01752 300250
www.digginit.org.uk
An organic community garden in Plymouth working with socially disadvantaged groups.

The Federation of City Farms and Community Gardens (FCFCG)
Bristol
0117 923 1800
www.farmgarden.org.uk

Incredible Edible Todmorden
Todmorden, Yorkshire
01706 815407
www.incredible-edible-todmorden.co.uk
A volunteer-run project that has transformed the small town of Todmorden in West Yorkshire into a place of edible abundance, with work including planting orchards, guerrilla veg gardening and collating a directory of local producers.

Transition Town Kinsale's Community Garden
www.transitiontownkinsale.org/projects/community-garden

The Whitehawk Community Food Project
Brighton
www.thefoodproject.org.uk

Websites

www.communitygarden.org
Website for the American Community Gardening Association.

www.guerrillagardening.org
Richard Reynolds' website with stories, films, photos and his blog.

www.moregardens.org
A New-York-based organisation that has had a number of amazing successes in protecting and nurturing community gardens in the city.

4 Community orchards

Books

Hogg, Robert (1884) *The Fruit Manual: A guide to the fruit and fruit trees of Great Britain*. Royal Horticultural Society.

King, Angela and Clifford, Sue (2008) *The Community Orchards Handbook*. Common Ground.

Morgan, Joan (2003) *The New Book of Apples*. Crown Publishing.

Sustain (2007) *Protecting Our Orchard Heritage*. Available at http://www.sustainweb.org/publications/info/162/

Organisations and projects

The Agroforestry Research Trust
See section 15 (General edible gardening) for contact details.

Common Ground
Shaftesbury, Dorset
01747 850820
www.commonground.org.uk

Donkey Field Community Orchard
Portobello, Edinburgh
http://pedal-porty.org.uk/food/orchard

Orchard Link
Totnes, Devon
07792 664710
www.orchardlink.org.uk
Supports orchard owners and workers with advice and encourages knowledge sharing and communication between orchards in its network.

Websites

http://www.england-in-particular.info/orchards/o-comm2.html
Webpage on Common Ground's England in Particular website about community orchards.

5 Community shops

Books

The Plunkett Foundation (2006) *Staff Handbook for a Community Owned Village Shop*. Available by contacting the organisation directly – see section 23 (Local food – general) for contact details.

Organisations and projects

Cooperatives UK
This organisation can assist groups wanting to set up community shops in urban areas. See section 12 (Food co-ops) for contact details.

Making Local Food Work
An initiative of the Plunkett Foundation. See section 23 (Local food – general) for contact details. See more about the Plunkett-Foundation-led Community Shops and Local Food project on www.makinglocalfoodwork.co.uk/about/cslf/index.cfm.

Rural Community Shops
The Plunkett Foundation's more general Rural Community Shops programme. See www.plunkett.co.uk/whatwedo/rcs/ruralcommunityshops.cfm, which has many advice sheets on setting up and running a community shop.

The Rural Shops Alliance
Weymouth, Dorset
01305 752044
www.rural-shops-alliance.co.uk

6 Community Supported Agriculture schemes (CSAs)

Books

Groh, Trauger and McFadden, Steven (1998) *Farms of Tomorrow Revisited: Community supported farms, farm supported communities*. Biodynamic Farming and Gardening Association.

Henderson, Elizabeth and Van En, Robyn (1999) *Sharing the Harvest: A guide to community supported agriculture.* Chelsea Green.

Junge, Sharon K., Ingram, Roger, Veerkamp, Garth E. and Blake, Bill (1995) *Community Supported Agriculture – Making the Connection: A 1995 handbook for producers.* University of California Cooperative Extension.

Organisations and projects

Canalside Community Food
Leamington Spa, Warwickshire
01926 423939
www.canalsidecommunityfood.org.uk

The Farnham Local Food Initiative (FLFI)
Farnham, Surrey
0844 415 2620
www.farnhamfood.com

Soil Association CSA team
0117 914 2424
http://www.soilassociation.org/Takeaction/Getinvolv-edlocally/Communitysupportedagriculture/tabid/201/Default.aspx
See section 23 (Local food – general) for main contact details of the Soil Association.

Stroud Community Agriculture Ltd
0845 458 0814
www.stroudcommunityagriculture.org

Websites

www.biodynamics.com/csa.html
An introduction to CSA from the Biodynamic Farming and Gardening Association.

www.featherstonefarm.com
A CSA based in Minnesota.

www.justfood.org/jf
A CSA based in New York City.

www.myfarmsf.com
An urban-based American CSA that operates from vegetable plots in back yards across cities.

www.sare.org/csa
Resources for producers and consumers from the US Sustainable Agriculture Research and Education.

7 Course centres

Bicton College
Devon
01395 562400
www.bicton.ac.uk

Garden Organic
See section 15 (General edible gardening) for contact details.

Growing Well
See section 23 (Local food – general) for contact details.

Naturewise
0845 458 4697
North London
www.naturewise.org.uk
Naturewise runs permaculture and forest-gardening workshops and courses.

Patrick Whitefield Associates
Glastonbury
01458 832317
www.patrickwhitefield.co.uk

Ragman's Lane Farm
Lydbrook, Gloucestershire
01594 860244
www.ragmans.co.uk

Spiralseed
Westcliff on Sea, Essex
www.spiralseed.co.uk
The permaculture teacher Graham Burnett's venture,

running courses and workshops (as well as selling a variety of books, CDs and DVDs).

8 Expanding local food projects

Organisations and projects

Growing Communities
London
020 7502 7588
www.growingcommunities.org

Other expanded and innovative local food projects mentioned elsewhere in this book include The Abundance Project Sheffield – see section 16 (Glut and gleaning), Incredible Edible Todmorden – see section 3 (Community gardens) and Organic Lea – see section 1 (Allotments).

9 Farmers' markets

Books

Chubb, Alan (1998) *Farmers' Markets – the UK potential*. Eco-logic Books.

Festing, Harriet (1998) *Farmers' Markets – an American Success Story*. Eco-logic Books.

Organisations and projects

Bath Farmers' Market
01761 490 624
www.bathfarmersmarket.co.uk

Country Markets Ltd (formerly Women's Institute Markets)
Chesterfield, Derbyshire
01246 261508
www.country-markets.co.uk

National Farmers' Retail and Markets Association (FARMA)
Winchester
0845 458 8420
www.farma.org.uk

Redland Farmers' Market
Sustainable Redland, Bristol
www.sustainableredland.org.uk

Wolverton farmers' market
Food Train, Wolverton, Milton Keynes
01908 221161
www.foodtrain.org.uk

Websites

www.farmersmarkets.net
FARMA's farmers' market website, with supportive tips, ideas and listings of member markets.

www.farmshopping.net
A website run by FARMA, showing locations of farmers' markets, farm shops, veg box schemes and so on.

10 Farming – general

Books

Harvey, Graham (1997) *The Killing of the Countryside*. Jonathan Cape.

Laughton, Rebecca (2008) *Surviving and Thriving on the Land: How to use your time and energy to run a successful smallholding*. Green Books.

Pretty, Jules (1998) *The Living Land – Agriculture, Food and Community Regeneration in Rural Europe*. Earthscan.

Schilthuis, W. (1994) *Biodynamic Agriculture*. Floris Books.

Farming and Wildlife Advisory Group (FWAG)
Kenilworth, Warwickshire
024 7669 6699
www.fwag.org.uk

Fordhall Organic Farm
Drayton, Shropshire
01630 638255
www.fordhallfarm.com
An organic farm that was famously saved from the threat of development when more than 8,000 members of the public purchased shares in what is now a community land initiative. The farm runs a number of events, courses and open days.

Land Heritage Trust
Exeter
01647 24511
www.landheritage.org.uk

National Farmers' Union (NFU)
Stoneleigh, Warwickshire
024 7685 8500
www.nfuonline.com

South Devon Community Supported Farming (CSF)
Harberton, Devon
01803 865631
www.greenlistings.co.uk/devoncsf

Tolhurst Organic Produce
Pangbourne, Berkshire
0118 984 3428
www.tolhurstorganic.co.uk
This farm runs a stock-free approach to organic farming. As well as running a local box scheme, Iain Tolhurst also runs an organic farming and growing consultancy service.

Women's Food and Farming Union
Stoneleigh, Warwickshire
0844 335 0342
www.wfu.org.uk

World Wide Opportunities on Organic Farms (WWOOF)
Winslow, Buckingham
www.wwoof.org.uk
This charity provides opportunities for volunteers to work on organic farms.

Websites

www.ncfi.org.uk
The National Care Farming Initiative: a national network providing supporting services for care farmers – farms providing social, educational and therapeutic opportunities.

www.soilassociation.org
There is a wealth of information on this website relating to organic agriculture. See section 23 (Local food – general) for main contact details.

11 Food and land mapping

Books

Clifford, Sue and King, Angela (eds.) (1996) *From Place to PLACE: Maps and parish maps*. Common Ground.

Organisations and projects

Geofutures
Bath
01225 788870
www.geofutures.co.uk

Websites

www.chickmappers.com/100miledietmap
A web map that applies the 100-mile-diet project (described in the Food Challenges section of Chapter 15, see page 117) to local food in Madison, USA.

www.greenmap.org
A website that allows you to develop maps of sustainable living in your area, currently being used by communities around the world.

www.makinglocalfoodwork.co.uk/about/fwm
This project is being run by CPRE to assist communities in mapping their own local food networks.

12 Food co-ops

Organisations and projects

Cooperatives UK
Manchester
0161 246 2900
www.cooperatives-uk.coop/live/cme0.htm

Food For All
Bristol
0117 964 7228
www.foodforallbristol.org.uk

Websites

www.foodcoops.org
Sustain's new food co-op website, complete with tools, tips and an online directory.

www.localfoodcoop.org
A website where you can download software for food co-op use.

www.oklahomafood.coop
The website of Robert Waldrop's food co-op in Oklahoma.

13 Funding, grants and loans

Biffaward
Newark, Nottinghamshire
01636 670000
www.biffaward.org
Grants for community and environmental projects across the UK using money from landfill tax credits donated by Biffa Waste Services.

The City Bridge Trust
London
020 7332 3710
www.bridgehousegrants.org.uk/CityBridgeTrust
Grants for projects benefiting the inhabitants of Greater London, including those for environmental education and for maintaining and enhancing London's biodiversity.

Community First
Devizes, Wiltshire
01380 722475
www.communityfirst.org.uk
Grants available for community projects in Wiltshire and Swindon.

Community Food and Health (Scotland)
Glasgow
0141 226 5261
www.communityfoodandhealth.org.uk
This government-funded organisation has grants available for community food projects in Scotland.

Community Spaces
Birmingham
0845 3671 671
www.community-spaces.org.uk
This lottery-funded grants programme, managed by Groundwork, supports community groups in creating or improving green spaces to enhance quality of life in neighbourhoods across England.

Cooperative and Community Finance
Bristol
0117 916 6750
www.icof.co.uk
Loans for cooperatives and social enterprises.

Deutsche Bank – Capital Community Foundation
London
020 7582 5117
www.capitalcf.org.uk/grants/grantsavailable.php
Grants intended to support groups working under the

themes of education and community development in the Camden, Lambeth, Lewisham and Westminster areas of London.

Esmée Fairbairn Foundation
London
020 7812 3700
www.esmeefairbairn.org.uk
This large grant-giving body now has a food-funding strand, prioritising the enjoyment and access of food (rather than its production), with a budget of £3 million over three years.

Futurebuilders England
A government-backed investment fund providing loans to charities and community-based organisations in England.
Newcastle
0191 261 5200
www.futurebuilders-england.org.uk

Green Prints
Falfield, Gloucestershire
01454 262910
www.sitatrust.org.uk/greenprints
This scheme, managed by the SITA Trust, offers grants for young people (aged 16-25) to improve green spaces for people and wildlife.

Heritage Lottery Fund
Find your local office on: www.hlf.org.uk/English/ContactUs/
Helpline: 020 7591 6000

j4b
www.j4b.co.uk
This organisation's website allows voluntary and community organisations to search for grants using its online database, but there is a subscription charge for all apart from the green and student-funding databases.

Lloyds TSB Foundation for England and Wales – Community Programme
London
0870 411 1223
www.lloydstsbfoundations.org.uk/FundingProgrammes/Pages/Community.aspx
This foundation supports small and medium charities that help disadvantaged people play a fuller role in the community.

Local Food
Newark, Nottinghamshire
0845 3671 671
www.localfoodgrants.org
These grants have been provided as part of the National Lottery's Changing Spaces programme. The decision has been taken, however, to bring the deadline for first stage applicants forward to August 2009.

Local Investment Fund
London
020 7680 1028
www.lif.org.uk
Loans for social and community enterprises across the UK.

Modernisation Fund
London
www.modernisationfund.org.uk/index.html
This fund is part of a government initiative to help third-sector organisations restructure and build resilience to meet the impact of the recession.

National Lottery Awards For All
0845 410 2030
www.awardsforall.org.uk
A lottery-funded grants scheme for small, local, community-based projects in the UK. See website for regional contact details.

Natural England – Access to Nature
0845 367 1671
www.naturalengland.org.uk/ourwork/enjoying/outdoorsforall/accesstonature/
This grant scheme aims to encourage people from all backgrounds to understand, access and enjoy the natural environment. The website gives further details of regional contacts.

O2 It's Your Community
0800 902 0250
www.itsyourcommunity.co.uk
O2 has teamed up with the Conservation Foundation to provide awards between £100 and £1,000 to projects that benefit local communities or that build community spirit.

Regional Development Agencies (RDAs)
These government-funded bodies provide grants for community-level projects and businesses, or, failing this, may be able to point you in the right direction of other appropriate sources of funding. In England there are nine RDAs, and there are also similar bodies in Scotland, Ireland and Wales.

England's RDAs
020 7222 8180
www.englandsrdas.com

Invest Northern Ireland
www.investni.com
See the website for contact details of regional offices.

Skills Development Scotland (SDS)
0141 225 6710
www.skillsdevelopmentscotland.co.uk

Welsh Development Agency
0845 010 3300 (English) 0845 010 4400 (Welsh)
www.wales.gov.uk/topics/businessandeconomy

Triodos Bank
Bristol
0117 973 9339
www.triodos.co.uk
This ethical bank helps to support a number of sustainability projects, including several that are focused on organic and local food work.

Trust for London
020 7606 6145
www.trustforlondon.org.uk
This independent charitable trust supports small, new and emerging voluntary organisations in London that work to improve the lives of people and communities in London.

Trusthouse Charitable Foundation
London
020 7264 4990
www.trusthousecharitablefoundation.org.uk
Grants available for non-profit-making organisations and community projects across the UK.

UnLtd
London
020 7566 1100
www.unltd.org.uk
Funding and support for social entrepreneurs to help realise their visions.

Voluntary Action Fund – Community Chest
Dunfermline, Fife
01383 620780
www.voluntaryactionfund.org.uk/grant-schemes/Comm
The Community Chest provides grants to voluntary and community-based organisations across Scotland.

14 Garden shares

Organisations and projects

Adopt-a-Garden scheme
Isle of Wight
01983 822282
www.footprint-trust.co.uk

Capital Growth
London
020 7837 1228
www.capitalgrowth.org

Landshare
www.landshare.net
Hugh Fearnley-Whittingstall's project, which matchmakes growers with landowners with spare land across the UK.

Tavistock Garden Share Alliance (TGSA)
Tavistock, Devon
01822 613743

Transition Town Totnes's Garden Share Project
Totnes, Devon
01803 867358
www.totnes.transitionnetwork.org/gardenshare/home

Websites

www.en-form.supanet.com/gardenshare.htm
The Colchester garden share register.

http://grow.transitionbrightonandhove.org.uk
Grow Your Neighbour's Own, a garden share scheme in
Brighton and Hove.

http://www.urbangardenshare.org
A US-based garden share project.

15 General edible gardening

Books and DVD

Crawford, Martin (1998) *Agroforestry Options for Landowners*.
Agroforestry Research Trust.

Crawford, Martin (2009) *A Forest Garden Year* (DVD). Green
Books.

Fern, Ken (1997) *Plants for a Future*. Permanent Publications.

Hamilton, Andy and Hamilton, Dave (2008) *The Self-
Sufficientish Bible*. Hodder & Stoughton.

Harrison, John (2008) *Vegetable Growing Month-by-Month*.
Right Way.

Larkcom , Joy (2008) *Creative Vegetable Gardening* (revised
edn). Mitchell Beazley.

Larkcom, Joy (2002) *Grow Your Own Vegetables*. Frances
Lincoln.

Whitefield, Patrick (1996) *How to Make a Forest Garden*.
Permanent Publications.

Organisations and projects

Agroforestry Research Trust (ART)
Totnes, Devon
01803 840776
www.agroforestry.co.uk
Martin Crawford's organisation, where you can buy plants,
seeds, publications and ART's quarterly journal.

Garden Organic
Coventry
024 7630 3517
www.gardenorganic.org.uk

The Good Gardeners Association
Wotton-under-Edge, Gloucestershire
01453 520322
www.goodgardeners.org.uk

Thrive
Reading
0118 988 5688
www.thrive.org.uk
This charity promotes and uses gardening as a therapy for
disabled people.

Websites

www.edibleforestgardens.com
Information on small-scale polyculture.

www.foodnotlawns.com
Project encouraging the use of gardens to grow food.

www.gardenbanter.co.uk
Gardening forum and newsgroup.

www.hedgewizardsdiary.blogspot.com
An informative and entertaining blog detailing one family's
experiences growing their own fruit and vegetables.

www.kitchengarden.co.uk
Website of *Kitchen Garden* magazine, with information, blog and forum.

www.selfsufficientish.com
Website and online community aimed at those who wish to produce more of their own food but do not have the resources to do so on a large scale, offering advice on allotments, growing vegetables, wild food and much more.

16 Glut and gleaning

Organisations and projects

Abundance Manchester
www.abundancemanchester.wordpress.com
The Manchester-based sister organisation of Abundance Sheffield.

The Abundance Project
Sheffield
www.growsheffield.com/pages/groShefAbun.html
Run by Grow Sheffield – see section 23 (Local Food – general) for contact details.

Websites

www.gleaningproject.org
A gleaning project that collects surplus food and distributes it to hungry people in Whatcom County, Washington, USA.

www.slowmovement.com/gleaning.php
A brief how-to guide to gleaning and food recovery.

17 The Great Reskilling

Books

Corbin, Pam (2008) *Preserves: River Cottage Handbook No.2*. Bloomsbury.

Fallon, Sally (1999) *Nourishing Traditions*. New Trends.

Fearnley-Whittingstall, Hugh (2003) *The River Cottage Cookbook*. Collins.

Gardeners and farmers of Terre Vivante (2007) *Preserving Food Without Freezing or Canning*. Chelsea Green.

Katz, Sandor (2006) *The Revolution Will Not Be Microwaved: Inside America's underground food movements*. Chelsea Green.

Katz, Sandor (2003) *Wild Fermentation: The flavor, nutrition, and craft of live-culture foods*. Chelsea Green.

Mabey, Richard (2007) *Food For Free* (revised edn). Collins.

Pitchford, Paul (2002) *Healing With Whole Foods: Asian Traditions and Modern Nutrition*. North Atlantic Books.

Ponsonby, Julia (2008) *Gaia's Kitchen*. Green Books.

Stevens, Daniel (2009) *Bread: River Cottage Handbook No.3*. Bloomsbury.

Warren, Piers (2008) *How to Store Your Garden Produce: The key to self-sufficiency*. Green Books.

Whitley, Andrew (2009) *Bread Matters: Why and how to make your own*. Fourth Estate Ltd.

Wright, John (2007) *Mushrooms: River Cottage Handbook No.1*. Bloomsbury.

Organisations and projects

Bread Matters
Penrith, Cumbria
01768 881899
www.breadmatters.com
Run by Andrew Whitely, this company holds courses, offers advice and supports producers of 'real bread'.

The No-Dig Gardening Project
www.transitionnelson.org.nz/no-dig-workshops

See sections 15 (General edible gardening) and 7 (Course centres) for more ideas.

Websites

http://poeticsofbread.blogspot.com
Eva Bakkeslett's bread blog.

www.schoolofeverything.com
A website where you can search for teachers or students (of almost anything) in your area.

www.sustainweb.org/realbread
The Real Bread Campaign's informative and helpful website with recipes, articles, a directory of 'real bread makers' and more.

www.vegbox-recipes.co.uk
Inspiration for cooking with seasonal vegetables.

www.wildfermentation.com
Sandor Katz's website.

www.wildmanwildfood.com
Fergus Drennan's website.

18 Home garden growing

Organisations and projects

Food Up Front
South London
07726 560703
www.foodupfront.org

Out of Our Own Back Yard
www.ooooby.ning.com
The New-Zealand-based Ooooby network of back-yard food growers.

Websites

www.growing-gardens.org
A US version of Food Up Front.

www.permablitz.net
An Australian website dedicated to the permablitzing approach to getting help in the home garden.

See section 15 (General edible gardening) for more resources.

19 Linking with local currencies

Books

Cato, Molly Scott (2006) *Market Schmarket*. New Clarion Press.

Organisations

LETS Link UK
London
www.letslinkuk.net

Websites

www.berkshares.org
The local currency for the Berkshire region of Massachusetts.

www.gaianeconomics.org
A website featuring writing by a group of economists, including Molly Scott Cato, who work to demystify the prevailing economic system.

www.ithacahours.org
The local currency used in Ithaca, New York.

www.thelewespound.org
The local currency for Lewes.

20 Local food challenges

Books

Kingsolver, Barbara (2008) *Animal, Vegetable, Miracle*. Faber and Faber.

Websites

http://100milediet.org
A challenge to eat food from within a 100-mile radius.

www.betheatslocal.org
Beth Tilston's blog about her challenge to eat only food from within 100 miles of her home in Brighton.

www.eatthechange.org
Website for the Eat the Change project, which calls people to eat local, organic, wild or plastic-free foods for a week.

www.fifediet.co.uk
A project that challenges people to eat food from the region of Fife.

21 Local food guides and directories

Websites

www.bigbarn.co.uk
Directory of local food suppliers. Also includes recipes and guides to what is in season.

www.eatlocalguide.com
Transition County Boulder's online local food directory.

www.hampshirefare.co.uk
Organisation promoting local producers in Hampshire.

www.herefordshirefoodlinks.org.uk
Directory of local producers in Herefordshire.

www.localfoodadvisor.com
Local food directory.

www.norwichfoodweb.org.uk
Network supporting community food projects in Norwich.

http://totnes.transitionnetwork.org/localfooddirectory/home
The webpage for Totnes's local food guide.

22 Local food events

Websites

www.thebiglunch.com
The website for the Eden project's nationwide Big Lunch idea, which encouraged people to get together with their neighbours and share their own home-grown and/or home-made food at neighbourhood street parties in July 2009.

www.realfoodfestival.co.uk
Website for London's Real Food Festival.

www.transitionnottingham.org.uk
Find out more about the urban harvest festival and other new projects on this initiative's website.

23 Local food – general

Books

De Selincourt, Kate (1997) *Local Harvest*. Lawrence Wishart.

Flores, Heather C. (2006) *Food Not Lawns: How to turn your lawn into a garden and your neighbourhood into a community.* Chelsea Green.

Halweil, Brian (2002) *Home Grown: The case for local food in a global market*. Worldwatch Institute.

Nabhan, Gary Paul (2002) *Coming Home to Eat: The pleasures and politics of local foods*. W. W. Norton & Co.

Norberg-Hodge, Helena, Merrifield, Todd and Gorelick, Steven (2002) *Bringing the Food Economy Home: Local alternatives to global agribusiness*. Kumarian Press.

Organisations and projects

Bristol Food Hub
www.bristolfoodhub.org
A small, not-for-profit organisation that works to empower communities to engage in sustainable forms of food production.

The Bulmer Foundation
Hereford
01432 294112
www.bulmerfoundation.org.uk

The Campaign to Protect Rural England (CPRE)
London
020 7981 2800
www.cpre.org.uk

East Anglia Food Links
Norwich
01508 536666
www.eafl.org.uk

Eat Somerset
www.sustainweb.org/eatsomerset
A project run by Sustain (see below for main contact details).

F3 – local food consultants
Bristol
0845 458 9525
www.localfood.org.uk

Food Futures Manchester
0161 234 4268
www.foodfutures.info

Food Matters
Brighton
01273 431707
www.foodmatters.org

Grow Sheffield
0114 258 0784
www.growsheffield.com

Growing Well
Kendal, Cumbria
01539 561777
www.growingwell.co.uk
An organic growing site and training centre.

The Land is Ours (TLIO)
South Petherton, Somerset
01460 249204
www.tlio.org.uk
Simon Fairlie's group that campaigns for land rights in the UK.

Local Action on Food
www.sustainweb.org/localactiononfood
Run by Sustain (see below for main contact details). Set up in 2008, this campaign builds on the work of the former Food Links UK. Paid members of the Local Action on Food network receive magazines, discounts on events, advice and support, and opportunities to link up with other local food projects around the country.

Making Local Food Work
www.makinglocalfoodwork.co.uk
This initiative is run by the Plunkett Foundation (see below) and shares the same telephone number.

The New Economics Foundation
London
020 7820 6300
www.neweconomics.org

The Plunkett Foundation
Woodstock, Oxfordshire
01993 810730
www.plunkett.co.uk

Skye Food Links
Skye and Lochalsh
01470 521293
www.tastelocal.co.uk/skye/foodlink

The Soil Association
Bristol
0117 314 5000
www.soilassociation.org

Somerset Community Food
Glastonbury, Somerset
01458 832983
www.somersetcommunityfood.org.uk

Sustain
London
020 7837 1228
www.sustainweb.org

The Wholesome Food Association
Hartland, Devon
01237 441118
www.wholesome-food.org.uk
An organisation that offers a cheaper, trust-based alternative to organic certification.

Women's Environmental Network (WEN)
London
020 7481 9004
www.wen.org.uk

Websites

www.cityfarmer.info
Organisation encouraging people to grow food in urban areas.

www.culiblog.org
Blog about food and food culture.

www.eatthesuburbs.org
Blog dedicated to adapting to peak oil and climate change in urban and suburban locations.

www.foodforchange.org.uk
Blog promoting sustainable, ethical and environmentally responsible food.

www.foodmapper.wordpress.com
A visual exploration of local food issues.

www.freerangereview.com
Local food community site where customers review suppliers.

www.freshideas.org.uk
A network supporting community food projects that aim to improve access to healthy / local food, particularly in disadvantaged areas.

www.ruaf.org
The website for the Ruaf Foundation (Resource Centres on Urban agriculture and Food security).

www.tasteofthewest.co.uk
One regional organisation dedicated to promoting local produce from and within the UK West Country.

www.thefutureoffood.com
A website dedicated to the insightful documentary of the same name.

24 Organisations giving financial, legal or organisational advice

Books

Horowitz, Shel (2000) *Grassroots Marketing: Getting noticed in a noisy world.* Chelsea Green.

Organisations and projects

Action with Communities in Rural England (ACRE)
Cirencester, Gloucestershire
01285 653477
www.acre.org.uk

Association of British Credit Unions Limited (ABCUL)
Manchester
0161 832 3694
www.abcul.org

Community Action Network (CAN)
London
www.can-online.org.uk
A charity that supports and guides social entrepreneurs and social enterprise initiatives.

Co-operatives UK
Manchester
0161 246 2900
www.cooperativesuk.coop

Development Trusts Association (DTA)
London
0845 458 8336
www.dta.org.uk

Groundwork
Birmingham
0121 236 8565
www.groundwork.org.uk
This charity works with communities and the private and public sectors on all aspects of community sustainability and regeneration across the UK.

Land Heritage Trust
Exeter
01647 24511
www.landheritage.org.uk

National Association of Credit Union Workers
Coventry
0845 456 2640
www.nacuw.org.uk

The Plunkett Foundation
See section 23 (Local food – general) for contact details.

Radical Routes
Leeds
0845 330 4510
www.radicalroutes.org.uk
A network of UK-based cooperatives working for positive social change.

UK Sustainable Investment and Finance Association
London
020 7749 9950
www.uksif.org

25 Producer collaboration

Websites

www.soilassociation.org
Contains information on how to link up with local producers. See section 23 (Local food – general) for main contact details.

www.stroudco.org.uk
Stroud Food Hub, an innovative new project linking consumers directly with producers. Consumers join the hub and are then able to order produce online from a variety of local producers, which is then collected at a weekly drop-off point..

26 Research

Organisations

Growing Well
See section 23 (Local food – general) for contact details.

Publications

The following are some examples of helpful papers and publications, available from the Soil Association and Sustain, to help kick-start the research process.

Soil Association (2001) *A Share in the Harvest – A Feasibility Study for Community Supported Agriculture.*

Soil Association (2007) *How to Set up a Vegetable Box Scheme.*

Soil Association (1998) *Local Food for Local People – A Guide to Local Food Links.*

Soil Association (2001) *Marketing Information for Organic Growers (Horticultural Crops) Fact Sheet.*

Soil Association (2000) *Organic Food and Farming Report 2000.*

Soil Association (2000) *The Biodiversity Benefits of Organic Gardening.*

Sustain (1999) *City Harvest: The feasibility of growing more food in London.*

Sustain (2008) *Growing Round the Houses.*

27 Seed, plant and food swaps

Books

Ashworth, Suzanne (2002) *Seed to Seed: Seed saving techniques for the vegetable gardener.* Seed Saver Publications.

Cherfas, Jeremy et al. (1996) *The Seed Saver's Handbook.* Grover Books.

Deppe, Carol (2000) *Breed Your Own Vegetable Varieties: The gardener's and farmer's guide to plant breeding and seed saving.* Chelsea Green.

Stickland, Sue (2008) *Back Garden Seed Saving: Keeping our vegetable heritage alive.* Eco-Logic Books.

Organisations and projects

Dyfi Valley Seed Savers
Machynlleth, Powys
www.dyfivalleyseedsavers.co.uk

Irish Seed Savers
Scariff, Co. Clare, Ireland
00 353 619 21866
www.irishseedsavers.ie

Seedy Sunday
info@seedysunday.org
www.seedysunday.org
The UK's biggest seed swap event, held annually in Brighton and Hove.

Websites

www.gardenorganic.org.uk/hsl
Webpage for the Heritage Seed Library at Garden Organic.

www.grain.org
Grain is a non-governmental organisation promoting sustainable agriculture and biodiversity.

www.growingcommunities.org/good-food-swap/index.htm
Growing Communities Good Food Swap, where people trade produce they have grown or made.

www.realseeds.co.uk
Suppliers of rare, heirloom or unusual non-hybrid seeds.

www.seedsavers.net
A network established in Australia to support and promote seed saving.

www.seedypeople.co.uk
A website that facilitates seed swapping across the UK.

28 School projects on local food

Books

Dyer, Alan and Hodgson, John (2003) *Let Your Children Go Back to Nature.* Capall Bann Publishing.

Murphy, Dominic (2008) *The Playground Potting Shed: A Foolproof Guide to Gardening with Children.* Guardian Newspapers Ltd.

Sykes, Rachel (2006) *Edible Gardens in Schools: A Growing Guide for Teachers.* Southgate Publishers.

Organisations and projects

Focus on Food
Halifax
01422 383191
www.focusonfood.org
This campaign is part of the Food For Life Partnership (see below), and works on bringing food education and cooking skills to schools in the UK.

Food For Life Partnership
c/o Soil Association
Bristol
0117 314 5180
www.foodforlife.org.uk

Health Education Trust
Alcester, Warwickshire
www.healthedtrust.com
Also a part of the Food For Life Partnership, this charity educates young people about issues of health and nutrition.

Websites

www.allotmentssouthwest.org.uk/gardeninginschools.htm
Advice and support for school gardens.

www.eco-schools.org.uk
Website for the Eco-Schools award programme, recognising schools' achievements in sustainability and environmental activity.

www.edibleplaygrounds.co.uk
A project that teaches children how to grow and cook vegetables.

www.foresteducation.org
Website for the Forest Education Initiative, which trains people to become forest school leaders, who encourage children to have a deeper understanding of forests and their place in the wider ecosystem.

www.growingschools.org.uk
A website designed to support teachers working with children of all ages in the 'outdoor classroom'.

www.naturewise.org.uk/page.cfm?pageid=nw-forest
Information on open and volunteer days at Naturewise's community forest. See section 7 (Course centres) for main contact details.

www.rhs.org.uk/schoolgardening
The Royal Horticultural Society's campaign to encourage more children to take up gardening.

www.sustainweb.org/childrensfoodcampaign
Sustain's children's food campaign.

29 The Transition movement

Books

Chamberlin, Shaun (2009) *The Transition Timeline: For a local, resilient future*. Green Books.

Hopkins, Rob (2008) *The Transition Handbook: From oil dependency to local resilience*. Green Books.

Organisations

The Transition Network
Totnes, Devon
01560 531882
www.transitionnetwork.org

Websites

www.transitionnetwork.org
The main website of the Transition movement.

www.transitionculture.org
The website of Rob Hopkins. The site is "An evolving exploration into the head, heart and hands of energy descent".

Below are the websites for the Transition initiatives included in this book, but there are many more besides! See 'official' initiatives listed on the Transition Network's website for more.

Portobello Transition Town
http://pedal-porty.org.uk

Sustainable Redland
www.sustainableredland.org.uk

Transition Boulder County, USA
www.bouldercountygoinglocal.com

Transition City Bath
www.transitionbath.org.uk

Transition City Bristol
www.transitionbristol.net

Transition City Canterbury
www.transitioncitycanterbury.blogspot.com

Transition City Nelson, New Zealand
www.transitionnelson.org.nz

Transition Leicester
www.transitiontowns.org/Leicester

Transition Nottingham
www.transitionnottingham.org.uk

Transition Town Brixton
www.site.transitiontownbrixton.org

Transition Town Bungay
www.transitiontowns.org/Bungay

Transition Town Glastonbury
www.transitiontowns.org/Glastonbury

Transition Town Kapiti, NZ
http://ttk.org.nz

Transition Town Kinsale
www.transitiontownkinsale.org

Transition Town Lewes
www.transitiontowns.org/Lewes
See also www.thelewespound.org

Transition Town Stroud
www.transitionstroud.org

Transition Town Totnes
www.totnes.transitionnetwork.org

Transition Town Tynedale
www.transitiontynedale.org

Transition Town Westcliff
www.westclifftransition.wordpress.com

Transition Town West Kirby
www.transitiontownwestkirby.org.uk

Transition Waiheke
www.transitiontowns.org.nz/waiheke
See also http://ooooby.ning.com

Transition Whitstable
www.transitionwhitstable.org.uk

30 Yet more sources of help and interest

Books

Burnett, Graham and Rimbaud, Penny (2006) *Earth Writings*. Spiralseed.

Burnett, Graham (2008) *Permaculture: A beginner's guide*. Spiralseed.

Schumacher, E. F. (1973) *Small is Beautiful: A study of economics as if people mattered*. Vintage.

Schwarz, Walter and Schwarz, Dorothy (1998) *Living Lightly: Travels in post-consumer society*. Jon Carpenter.

Whitefield, Patrick (1993) *Permaculture in a Nutshell*. Permanent Publications.

Whitefield, Patrick (2004) *The Earth Care Manual*. Permanent Publications.

Organisations and projects

BTCV
Doncaster
01302 388883
www2.btcv.org.uk
A charity that runs a wide variety of environmental conservation projects across the UK, with many opportunities for volunteering and training.

The Department for the Environment, Food and Rural Affairs (Defra)
Customer Contact Unit: 0845 933 5577
www.defra.gov.uk

Food Ethics Council
Brighton
0845 345 8574
www.foodethicscouncil.org

Friends of the Earth
London
020 7490 1555
www.foe.co.uk

Greenpeace
London
020 7865 8100
www.greenpeace.org.uk

Natural England
Sheffield
0845 600 3078
www.naturalengland.org.uk
Statutory body advising the government on issues concerning the natural environment, including farming, conservation and the protection of wildlife.

Permaculture Association
London
0845 458 1805
www.permaculture.org.uk

Sustainable Living Initiative
Norwich
www.grow-our-own.co.uk

The Wildlife Trusts
Newark, Nottinghamshire
01636 677711
www.wildlifetrusts.org

Websites

www.communitysolution.org
A resource for low-energy living and education about climate change and peak oil.

www.ecolots.co.uk
An environmentally friendly free ad service.

www.enviromantics.com
A blog about sustainability, especially food systems and diets.

www.darkoptimism.org
The website of Shaun Chamberlin, author of *The Transition Timeline: For a local, resilient future*.

www.uk.freecycle.org
The website for the UK-wide network of freecyclers, who offer items free to other group members. Can be a helpful source of gardening equipment.

www.globalideasbank.org/site/home
A website showcasing innovative ideas and projects, posted by readers.

www.sharonastyk.com
An inspiring and informative blog about peak oil and how we can prepare for it.

www.towns.org.uk
The Action for Market Towns' website, promoting regeneration for market towns across the UK.

www.yesterdaysfuture.net
A blog by James Samuel of Transition Island Waiheke, New Zealand.

INDEX

Abundance Manchester 169, 201
ABUNDANCE project, London 87-8
Abundance project, Sheffield 169, 201
Adopt-a-Garden, Isle of Wight 72, 199
agrochemicals 15
    see also fertilisers and pesticides
agroforestry see forest gardens
allotments 12, 15, 47, 56-69
    historical background 57
    plot size 56
    privately owned 56, 58
    productivity 56
    rents 56
    resources 190-1
    selling produce 56, 69
    shared plots 56
    statutory allotments 56
    temporary allotments 56
    UK numbers of 56
    waiting lists 47, 57
    see also community allotments;
        community gardens; garden
        shares
Allotments Regeneration Initiative
    191
Ambridge (The Archers) 14
Anderson, Teresa 181
Andrews, Peter 115, 116, 117
animal husbandry 23
Apple Day 91-2
apples 12, 45, 92, 154
Arkwright, Richard 66, 67, 68

Awaiting Allotment Society, West Kirby
    58-9, 191

back gardens see home garden growing
Baines, Tim 95-6, 98
Bakkeslett, Eva 39
Balfour, Lady Eve 20
Barry, Caroline 86, 87
Bashford, Jade 106
Bath Farmers' Market 115-17, 188, 195
Berry, Wendell 7
biodiesel 111
biodynamic growing 24, 63, 159, 161,
    186
Blue Peter 17
Blunos, Martin 137
Bomford, Michael 20
bottling 45
box schemes 17, 79, 103, 127, 128, 145,
    159, 160, 161, 163
Boycott, Rosie 10
Boyle, Mark 171
bread and bread making 39, 40-1
Bristol and District Market Gardeners
    Association 11, 18
Britain
    ability to feed itself 15, 17
    future food system for 15, 17, 18-19,
        105
Broadlands Community Orchard,
    Bathford 95-6, 117
Brook, Joel 112

Brown, Julie 17, 159
Brown, Lou 74, 75, 76, 78
Brownlee, Michael 138, 139
Burnett, Graham 49, 50

Campaign to Protect Rural England
    (CPRE) 166, 204
Campbell, Margaret 58-9, 68
Canalside Community Food,
    Leamington Spa 22, 109-11, 194
canning 45
Capital Growth, London 10, 72, 199
carbon emissions 15
    sources 23
    UK government target 15
carbon sinks 15
A Celebration of Local Food (Totnes)
    134-6
Chamberlin, Shaun 31, 47
children
    engaging 10, 66, 141, 142
    school meals 141-2
    see also school projects on local food
cider making 92
city farms 17
Clifford, Sue 94
climate change 13, 21
    tipping points 13
comfort zones, moving beyond 28-9
Common Ground 91, 94, 193
communication channels 32, 33, 179-83
    see also publicity

community allotments 56-7, 69
   challenges and rewards 59, 61-2, 64-5
   projects 58-67
   tips 68-9
   see also community gardens
community assistance, offers of 30, 110, 112, 178
community cafes and restaurants 174
community composting 164-5, 191-2
community gardens 56-7, 79-90
   challenges and rewards 64, 82, 85, 87-8
   guerilla gardening 80, 81, 178, 192
   historical background to 79
   projects 84-9
   resources 192-3
   school projects 143-4
   tips 90
   UK numbers of 79
   see also community allotments
community groups, defining 27-8
community orchards 66, 91-101, 160
   challenges and rewards 92, 94
   events 92, 94, 95
   fruit storage 100
   glut and gleaning projects 169-70
   health and safety issues 100
   new orchards 92, 100
   practicalities 92
   produce 92, 93
   projects 95-8
   resources 193
   timber 93
   tips 98, 99
community shops 165, 193
community space, opening up 27-8
Community Supported Agriculture (CSA) 102-13
   background to 102-3
   core principles 103

financial benefits 103
funding 107, 112
organic and biodynamic principles 103, 105
projects 106-11
resources 193-5
shareholders 105, 107-8
tips on setting up a CSA 112-13
composting 164-5, 191-2
consumerism 11, 13
cooking and food preparation 37-8, 39, 40-1, 42, 44-5
Cooper, Rob 38
cooperative approach 123
   see also food cooperatives
Cooperatives UK 165, 193, 197
coppicing 111
Council for the Protection of Rural England (CPRE) 183
council waste-collection schemes 164
Country Markets 114-15, 195
   see also farmers' markets
Countryside Agency 118
course centres 194-5
Crawford, Ingrid 85-7, 90
Crawford, Martin 99, 143
creativity 29
Cuban organic food-growing revolution 47
Culhane, Anne-Marie 169
currencies, local 52, 135, 170-1, 202

Dalmeny, Kath 125
Daniel, Amanda 105
data harvesting 179, 181
Davies, Clare 152, 153, 156
De Selincourt, Kate 132, 133
decision-making
   good information, accessing 31
   shared 28, 103, 108, 123, 131
Defra 12, 164

dehydrators 45
Denzer, Kiko 39
Dig for Victory campaign (WWII) 12, 65
Diggers movement 79
diversity 15
   promoting 33
Dobma, Doeke 155-6
Don, Monty 147
Donkey Field Community Orchard, Portobello, Edinburgh 96-7, 193
Downs, Georgina 27
Drennan, Fergus 37, 40-1, 171
dried foods 45
Dunwell, Matt 132, 133

East Anglia Food Links 155, 204
Eastwood Comprehensive School 147-8
Eat the Change initiative 171, 182, 203
Eat Local Resource Guide and Directory (Colorado, USA) 138-9
Eat Somerset 182, 204
edible landscaping as art form 17
elder community, involving 35-6, 178
Energy Descent Action Plan (EDAP) 180, 183, 189
energy efficiency 111
ethics of care 123
expanding local food projects 158-63, 195

F3 21, 204
fair trade 162
Fairlie, Simon 17, 166, 167
farmers' markets 114-22
   challenges and rewards 117, 119, 121
   criteria 114
   funding 120-1
   local traders, working with 121, 122

organisation 117, 118-19
projects 115-21
resources 195
site requirements 121-2
tips 121-2
UK numbers of 114
see also Country Markets
farming
'carbon positive' 13, 15
future vision for 15
livestock 16
mixed 16
producer-consumers 17
resources 195-6
in transition 26
wartime productivity 12
see also Community Supported
Agriculture (CSA); farmers'
markets; food cooperatives
Farnham Local Food Initiative 112
Fearnley-Whittingstall, Hugh 73, 76
Federation of City Farms and Community Gardens (FCFCG) 79, 82,
95, 183
fermentation 42
fertilisers and pesticides 15, 23, 27, 186
Fife food challenge 171-2, 203
financial advice 205-6
Focus on Food 146, 207
food calendars 174
food cooperatives 123-31
buying in food 127-8
challenges and rewards 127-8,
129-30
collection points 129, 131
projects 124-30
publicity 129
recruiting customer-members 130
resources 197
tips 130-1
web-based 130

Food Ethics Council 183
food feet 12, 41, 67
Food For All, Hartcliffe, Bristol 124-6,
197
Food For Life Partnership 145-8, 161,
208
food guides and directories 116, 132-40
advertising space 140
compilation tips 139-40
definitions and boundaries 132, 135
funding 135, 137, 140
projects 134-9
resources 203
food and land mapping 166-9, 180,
181, 182, 183, 196-7
Food Links UK 21
Food Matters 21, 204
food miles 12, 22, 23, 41, 49, 74, 102,
126, 128
food philosophies 24
food security 12, 57, 77, 120, 131
Defra view on 12
national decline of 12
reskilling for 35, 36
food swap events 173, 207
Food Train 118, 119, 120
Food Up Front, London 53-4, 202
food zones 16, 17
food-growing approaches 24
foodsheds 20, 23, 185
foraging 37, 40-1
Forest Food Directory (Forest of Dean)
132, 133
forest gardens 24, 92, 99, 142-4, 186
resources 200-1
Former LETS Allotment project,
Stroud 62-5
fossil-fuel dependence 11, 20, 26, 82,
105, 111, 125
fruit imports 91
Fruit and Veg Together Co-op, Milton,

Westcliff 126-8
Fuller, Buckminster 29
funding, grants and loans
resources 17, 177, 197-9
see also financial advice

Garden Organic 110, 146, 183, 200
Garden Share Alliance, Tavistock 72
Garden Share Project, Totnes 74-6
garden shares 71-8
projects 74-7
resources 199-200
rewards 75-6
sharing arrangements 72, 74-5, 78
tips 78
garden tours 50-1
gardens *see* allotments; community
gardens; garden shares; home
garden growing
genetically modified crops 15
Geofutures 166, 183, 196
geographic information science (GIS)
166-7
Glastonbury Community Garden 85-7
Glastonbury Local Food Directory 136-8
global economic slowdown 13, 21
glut and gleaning projects 169-70, 201
Good Food Swap events 160
Goverd, Keith 117
green manures 63, 110
greenhouse gases 10, 15, 23, 164
Grow Food Not Lawns, USA 36
Grow Sheffield 169, 204
Growing Communities, London 17,
22, 119, 158-63, 179, 195
core principles 161-3
food zones model 16, 17
outreach work 160-1, 179
trading systems 159-60
urban food production 160
growing food, pleasures of 18

Growing Local Conference, Bungay 154-6
Growing Well 173, 204
guerilla gardening 80, 81, 178, 192

Hansen, James 13
Harris, Louise 126, 127
Hart, Robert 143
Hartcliffe Health and Environment Action Group (HHEAG) 124-5, 126
Harvest Inspiration, Leicester 153-4
healing powers of gardening 86
Health Education Trust 146, 208
Healthy Start vouchers 128
Heinberg, Richard 20, 48
Hemming, Frank 98
Hepworth, Ruth 147
Holden, Patrick 26
Holmes, Sue 75-6
home garden growing 12, 15, 17, 19, 47-55
    Cuban food-growing revolution 47
    engaging community members 55
    projects 49-55
    resources 202
    tips 49, 55
    UK potential for feeding people 71
    see also allotments
Hopkins, Rob 10, 11-19, 84
horses, working 109, 112

inclusion and openness 31-2
Incredible Edible Todmorden 80, 192
information, enabling access to 31
Ingall, Tom and Caz 109, 110, 111, 113

jam making 44-5
Jones, Bob 36-7, 46

Katz, Sandor Ellix 42
Kiddey, Nick 97, 98

King, Eleanor 127, 128, 130
Kingsolver, Barbara 171
Kinsale's Transition Community Garden 84-5, 192

Land Trusts 79, 188
landfills 164
Landshare 73, 76, 199
Law, Duncan 87, 88, 90
legal advice 205-6
Lewis, Caroline 137, 139
Litherland, Ru 156
Local Action on Food 21, 204
Local Exchange Trading Systems (LETS) 62-3, 187
local food challenges 171-2, 202-3
local food culture 12, 18-19
    brought-in food 22
    criteria and definitions 21-3
    local food boundaries 22
    rewards 153
    shift towards 20-1
    urban-based, low-carbon culture 16
local food events 150-7
    ideas for 156, 174
    projects 151-6
    publicity 151, 152-3
    resources 203
    themed 150
    tips 151, 156-7
    venues 151
Local Food Fund 17
local food networks
    building 21, 180-1
    economics-based assessment 23
    growth of 21
    social benefits 23
local food projects
    alternatives, building 29-30
    comfort zones, moving beyond 28-9
    creating 175-84

data harvesting 179, 181
elder community, involving 178
forming a group 33, 175-6
funding 177
help, enlisting 178
legal issues 177
networking 176
planning 177
project, choosing 176-7
project growth 178
publicity 178-9
creativity 29
expanding 158-63, 195
linking projects 180
outreach work 160-1, 179-80
place, reconnection with 29
principles
    inclusion and openness 31-2
    information, enabling access to 31
    nurturing environment 33-4
    positive visioning 30-1, 177
    resilience, building 32-3
    sharing and networking 32
    subsidiarity 34
shared decision-making 28
shared ownership 28
'sowing and reaping' 30, 110, 178
'locavores' 22, 171
Lujic, Zoe 53

Macbeth, Sheila 63, 64, 65, 68
Mackenzie, Noni 134, 135, 139
MacKinnon, James 171
Making Local Food Work programme 21, 165, 166, 193, 204
Manchester City Council parks 17
mapping exercises 166-9, 180, 181, 182, 183
market gardens 11, 160

see also community allotments; community gardens
Master Chef Series, Whitstable 37-8
Mayfield, Seb 53, 54
meat eating 15, 17, 24, 188
Meldrum, Josiah 155, 156
Mellanby, Kenneth 15, 17
Menzies, Ross 145, 148
methane 23, 164
Michael, Lisa 154, 156
Miliband, Ed 14
Milne, Claire 182, 183
Milton Community Partnership 126-7
mulching 36, 69
multilateral engagement and communication 27
Murray, Abi 37, 38, 46

National Farmers' Retail and Market Association (FARMA) 114
National Lottery funding 135, 198
National Trust 58
Naturewise 143
Naturewise Community Forest Garden, London 142-4
networking, enabling 32, 176
New Economics Foundation 183, 204
nitrogen fertilisers 13
nitrous oxide 23
No-Dig Gardening Project, New Zealand 36-7, 201
non-judgemental principle 34
Nottingham Urban Harvest Festival 151-3
Nunis, Thalia 110

Obama, Michelle 82
oil
    oil-free vision 14, 30
    peak oil 10, 13, 14, 21
Oklahoma food co-op 130, 197

Open Kitchen Gardens Project, Lewes 50-1
Open Orchard Project, New Zealand 97-8, 169
Open Space Technology 77, 134, 156, 180, 187-8
oral heritage project 67
orchards
    loss of 91
    see also community orchards
organic certification 103, 177
Organic Lea, London 57, 169, 191
organic methods and produce 23, 24, 26, 65, 103, 105, 119, 146, 159, 160, 161, 186, 196
organisational advice 205-6
Out Of Our Own Back Yard, New Zealand 51-2, 202
outreach work 160-1, 179-80
ownership, shared 28, 54, 55, 88, 90, 108, 112, 123, 131, 140, 165

Patchwork Farm Project, London 160
peak oil 10, 13, 14, 21
Pemberton, Alissa 118, 119
Permablitizing, Australia 54, 202
permaculture 24, 47, 49, 54, 84, 186
Permaculture Association 183
Pfeiffer, Dale Allen 11
place, reconnection with 29
plant swap events 173, 207
Playground Veg Stall, Tynedale 144-5
Plunkett Foundation 21, 165, 204
Ponsonby, Julia 44-5
Portobello Energy Descent and Land Reform Group (PEDAL) 96
positive visioning 30-1, 177
preserving foods 44-5
producer–consumer collaboration 172, 183, 206
publicity 32, 113, 129, 151, 178-9

raffles 46
raised beds 36
Rankine, Kerry 163
Real Bread Campaign 39
reconnecting with food 18-19, 20, 171
Redland Farmers' Market, Bristol 120-1, 195
Regan-Jones, Holly 128-9, 130
research projects 172-3, 206-7
resilience 12, 15, 124, 186-7
    building 32-3, 69, 85, 103, 129
    organising for 33
reskilling 35-46, 72, 105
    projects 36-8
    reskilling events, tips for 46
    tutelage 35-6
    workshops, ideas for 38-45
resources 190-210
Reynolds, Richard 81, 178
River Nene organic box scheme 127, 128
Robert Barton Trust 86
Roosevelt, Eleanor 82
Rundle-Keswick, Andrew 77, 78
Rural Community Shops Association 165, 193
rural landscape 15
Russell, Pete 51-2, 55

St Ann's Allotments, Nottingham 65-7, 191
Schonveld, Eva 96, 98
school local food projects 141-9
    projects 142-8
    resources 207-8
    rewards 143-4, 145, 148
    safety issues 149
    tips 148-9
School Nutrition Action Group (SNAG) 146, 147
Scrannage, Lin 74

Scrumping Project, Waltham Forest 169
Second World War 12, 57
seed banks 180
seed sales 47
seed swap events 61, 173
    resources 207
self-organisation 34
self-reliance 17, 27
Senter, Polly 50, 55
sharing, enabling 32, 33
shopping habits 20-1
Siveyer, Kathryn 60, 61, 68
skills development 78, 82, 83, 105
    resources 201-2
Skye Food Links 21, 204
Smith, Alissa 171
Sneed, Catherine 86
social relationships, strengthening of
    23, 29, 58
Soil Association 21, 26, 105, 146, 172,
    183, 204
    sustainable food plan for Britain 105
soil building 15
soil management 15, 36
Solnit, Rebecca 24-5
Somerset Food Links 137
'sowing and reaping' 30, 110, 178
Spriggs, James 147, 148
Stagg, Bethan 90
Starter Farm Project, London 160
Stoke Newington Farmers' Market
    159-60
Stroud Community Agriculture 22,
    103, 106-9, 194
Stroud Slad Farm Community 107
subsidiarity 34
sugar 44, 45
sun-dried fruits and vegetables 45
Sustain 21, 39, 125, 166, 183, 205
Sustainable Bungay 155, 156
Sustainable Redland 120, 121

swapping events 61, 160, 173, 207
Swatridge, Kate 53, 54, 55

Thurstain-Goodwin, Mark 166-7
Tilston, Beth 171, 203
timber 17, 93
Tolhurst, Iain 110
Torgut, Alpay 143
Transition City Allotment, Canterbury
    59-62
Transition City Bath 96, 117
Transition City Bristol 98, 126, 182
Transition City Canterbury 60
Transition City Leicester 154
Transition City Nottingham 67, 152
Transition City Stroud 62
Transition Handbook 35, 175, 208
Transition movement 14-15, 18, 24, 26
    building alternatives 29
    consultancy 14
    environmental factors, and pressure
        for change 13-14
    Food Strategy 183
    food web portal 183
    Great Reskilling 35
    initiatives 14, 24
    principles 30-4
    resources 208-9
    role of 14
    Transition training 14
Transition Primer 175
Transition Timeline 31, 47, 208
Transition Town Brampton 173
Transition Town Kapiti 77
Transition Town Kinsale 84, 142
Transition Town Leamington Spa 111
Transition Town Lewes 50, 170
Transition Town Stroud 108
Transition Town Totnes 74, 98, 134,
    166, 167, 168-9, 170, 172, 181
Transition Town Wellington 128

Transition Town Westcliff 126
Transition Town Whitstable 37
Transition Town Wolverton 120
transparency 31, 103, 132, 161
Travelling Garden Group, New
    Zealand 35, 76-7
trust 31, 33, 72, 103, 105, 108

Urb Farm, Wolverton 119
Urban Food Growing network, London
    53

Virtual Orchard Initiative, Bristol 98
volunteers, engaging 31, 113

Wakeman, Tully 155
Waldrop, Robert 130
Walker, Sue 126, 130
water usage 15
Watts, Stephen 169
Weir, Nick 108
Wellington Food Cooperative 128-30
Weymouth, Ray 129
White, Claire 143, 144, 148
Whitefield, Patrick 83, 85
Whitehawk Community Food Project,
    Brighton 84, 88-9, 192
Wholesome Food Association 135, 205
wild food see foraging
Wilkie, Jim 120, 121
Wills, Hamish 120
Winstanley, Gerard 79, 82
Wolverton Farmers' Market 117-20, 195
Women's Institute (WI) 114-15
    see also Country Markets
Wood, Jonny 120, 121
Wright, Daniel 58-9

Zev Benn, Dan 84-5, 90